Antisocial and Violent Youth

Volume II

The latest research in an easy-to-read format

EDITORS:

Jalal Shamsie, MB, FRCPC, FRCPsych
Professor of Psychiatry, University of Toronto
Director, Institute for the Study of Antisocial Behaviour in Youth
Staff Psychiatrist, Centre for Addiction and Mental Health

Joanne Lawrence, BA
Institute for the Study of Antisocial Behaviour in Youth
Centre for Addiction and Mental Health

Carole Hood, PhD
Institute for the Study of Antisocial Behaviour in Youth
Centre for Addiction and Mental Health

FOREWORD BY:

David P. Farrington, PhD
Professor of Psychological Criminology
Cambridge University, England

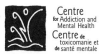

Centre
for Addiction and
Mental Health
Centre de
toxicomanie et
de santé mentale

A Pan American Health Organization /
World Health Organization
Collaborating Centre

Antisocial and Violent Youth · Volume II
The latest research in an easy-to-read format

National Library of Canada Cataloguing in Publication

Antisocial and violent youth, volume II /
edited by Jalal Shamsie, Joanne Lawrence and Carole Hood.

Includes index.

ISBN 0-88868-435-5

1. Conduct disorders in adolescence. 2. Violence in adolescence.
I. Shamsie, Jalal II. Lawrence, Joanne III. Hood, Carole (Carole Louise), 1945–
IV. Centre for Addiction and Mental Health

HQ799.2.V56A573 2003   616.85'82'00835   C2003-900075-3

Printed in Canada

For information on other Centre for Addiction and Mental Health
resource materials or to place an order, please contact:

Marketing and Sales Services
Centre for Addiction and Mental Health
33 Russell Street
Toronto, Ontario
Canada M5S 2S1

Tel.: 1 800 661-1111 or 416 595-6059 in Toronto

E-mail: marketing@camh.net

Web site: www.camh.net

This book was produced by:

Development
Margaret Kittel Canale, M.Ed., CAMH

Editorial
Sue McCluskey, CAMH

Design
Bob Tarjan, CAMH

Production
Christine Harris, CAPPM, CAMH

2741 / 03-03   PR057

Foreword

I am delighted to welcome this book as an exceptionally important contribution to understanding antisocial and violent behaviour in youth. It is a wonderful resource not only for busy practitioners and policy-makers but also for busy scholars and researchers. The contents are remarkably wide-ranging, covering risk and protective factors as well as prevention and treatment techniques for an extensive variety of problems in childhood and adolescence: delinquency, aggression, violence, conduct disorder, ADHD, substance use problems and suicide. All those who read this book will learn a great deal about the frontiers of knowledge in the field of childhood and adolescent psychopathology.

Dr. Jalal Shamsie should be warmly congratulated for at least three great achievements. First, he started to publish the newsletter *Youth Update* 20 years ago and is still publishing it today. *Youth Update* is an extremely valuable resource that contains summaries of the most up-to-date research findings, selecting clinically relevant articles from over 70 professional journals. *Youth Update* is particularly important in fostering evidence-based practice because the information and how it is presented can be easily understood by practitioners. Deservedly, it is now internationally famous.

Second, Dr. Shamsie had the brilliant idea of collecting these summaries of research findings into a single organized volume called *Antisocial and Violent Youth*. This book, now known as Volume I, was published to critical acclaim in 1999. It covered the period from the founding of *Youth Update* in 1983 up to 1997.

Third, Dr. Shamsie has now produced the present update, Volume II, which covers the period from 1997 to 2002. Like Volume I, it is a great resource.

How has knowledge about antisocial and violent youth advanced? I have not carried out a systematic analysis of Volume II, but here are my impressions after reading it. First, there have been enormous advances in knowledge about risk and protective factors, mainly derived from large-scale public health surveys and continuing longitudinal surveys of antisocial behaviour. Virtually all the major surveys can be found in either Volume I or Volume II. Second, knowledge about effective methods of prevention and treatment, based on high-quality experimental evaluations, is rapidly increasing. Again, most of the major intervention studies can be found in either Volume I or Volume II. Fortunately, many of these evaluations show that there are effective methods that may significantly reduce the damage to society caused by antisocial behaviour. The challenge to researchers is to communicate effectively about what works—not only to practitioners but also to government policy-makers and the media—and this book should help a great deal in achieving this aim.

As might have been expected, new studies about risk and protective factors, and prevention and treatment methods are the latest advancements. However, this volume also shows that more efforts are being made to link fundamental and applied research by using the results of risk- and protective-factor studies to improve intervention methods. This was also an aim of Rolf Loeber and myself in our two recent edited volumes (Loeber & Farrington, 1998, 2001). Ideally, evaluations of the effectiveness of intervention techniques should also teach us about risk and protective factors; however, this has not yet happened to any great degree, mostly because intervention techniques use a variety of approaches, and it is difficult to isolate the effects of their different ingredients.

It seems there is more research on bullying and on the effectiveness of school-based programs in this volume, no doubt reflecting the increased importance of these topics. Also, there were more summaries of systematic reviews and meta-analyses of intervention studies. The Campbell Collaboration was recently founded to carry out systematic reviews of the effectiveness of intervention programs and to make these reviews available to everyone through the Internet (Farrington & Petrosino, 2001).

This volume is a wonderful resource of up-to-date information about influencing factors and effective interventions for antisocial behaviour in childhood and adolescence. It is also easily readable. I am delighted to recommend this volume, together with Volume I, as essential reading for scholars and practitioners who are concerned with antisocial and violent behaviour in youth.

David P. Farrington, PhD
Professor of Psychological Criminology
Cambridge University, England.

REFERENCES

Farrington, D.P. & Petrosino, A. (2001). The Campbell Collaboration Crime and Justice Group. *Annals of the American Academy of Political and Social Science, 578,* 35–49.

Loeber, R. & Farrington, D.P. (Eds.). (1998). *Serious and Violent Juvenile Offenders: Risk Factors and Successful Interventions.* Thousand Oaks, CA: Sage.

Loeber, R. & Farrington, D.P. (Eds.). (2001). *Child Delinquents: Development, Intervention, and Service Needs.* Thousand Oaks, CA: Sage.

Contents

Chapter 4:
Attention-Deficit Hyperactivity Disorder   121

Chapter 5:
Juvenile Offenders   143

Chapter 6:
Abuse and Neglect   167

Introduction

Volume I of *Antisocial and Violent Youth* provided a review of the literature related to youth antisocial behaviour published in scientific journals from 1983 to 1997. This volume covers the period from 1997 to 2002. We were very gratified by the excellent reviews that the first volume earned, which have encouraged us to continue to provide in book format easy-to-read abstracts of the clinically relevant literature related to the subject of anti-social youth.

Our goal remains to promote evidence-based practice for professionals who work with youth who are antisocial. We realize that even with the best intentions it is not easy for professionals to keep abreast of the latest developments in the field. Research related to antisocial behaviour appears in over 70 professional journals. Most of the papers appearing in journals are written in technical language—readers need sophisticated knowledge in research methodology to understand it. Most professionals, childcare workers, social workers, probation officers and others in the field do not have the time or resources to benefit from the latest advances in the field. It was this realization that led to the publication of the newsletter *Youth Update* 20 years ago, providing abstracts, selected from journals, written in an easy-to-read format. Volume II, like Volume I, is a compilation of abstracts that appeared in *Youth Update*.

Each chapter is divided into sections according to a major line of study:

- characteristics and related issues
- etiology (causes)
- prevention
- treatment.

We believe that this volume includes most of the significant contributions made in the field in the last five years.

Jalal Shamsie, Joanne Lawrence, Carole Hood

Chapter 1
Antisocial Behaviour

Antisocial Behaviour

All criminal behaviours that are not indicted, and all behaviours that are not criminal but deviate from major social norms (e.g., compulsive lying, running away, truancy [not attending school]).

By definition this entire book pertains to antisocial behaviour. This chapter includes abstracts that do not specifically fit into any of the other chapters, but instead pertain to antisocial behaviours generally or to specific groups that may be perceived as antisocial (e.g., gangs).

Characteristics and Related Issues

Dangerously Violent Adolescents

Despite the decreased rates of homicides committed by adolescents, adolescents are responsible for a significant percentage of crime and violence. Studies have shown that there is a consistent relationship between being the victim of violence and commiting violent acts.

A sample of dangerously violent (DV) adolescents, who reported attacking someone with a knife or shooting at someone in the past year, was compared with a matched community sample of non-violent adolescents (control group).

RESULTS

- DV adolescents reported higher levels of exposure to violence and victimization than their non-violent counterparts.

- DV adolescents were two to four times more likely than children in control groups to have hit, beaten up and threatened someone in the past year.

- DV females were three to five times more likely to show clinical levels of all trauma symptoms (anger, anxiety, depression, dissociation, post-traumatic stress) than female controls.

- One in five DV females was at high risk for suicide.

- DV males were one to three times more likely to exhibit clinical levels of anger, dissociation and post-traumatic stress.

- DV males were three to six times more likely to have been a victim or witness of violence than were male controls.

COMMENT

This study, conducted on school populations, highlights the importance of adequately assessing students who have been exposed to violence and psychological trauma and giving them and their families adequate help.

SOURCE

Flannery, D.J., Singer, M.I. & Wester, K. (2001). Violence exposure, psychological trauma, and suicide risk in a community sample of dangerously violent adolescents. *Journal of the American Academy of Child and Adolescent Psychiatry, 40*(4), 435–442.

Psychiatric Disorders in Children Involved in Bullying

In this study the total sample consisted of 6,017 children with a mean age of 8.4 years. Researchers found that 5.7 per cent were bullies, 18.6 per cent were bully-victims (they bullied and were bullied themselves) and 24.8 per cent were victims (they were victims of bullying but did not bully others).

RESULTS

- Among bullies, 29.2 per cent had attention-deficit disorder, 12 per cent experienced depression and 12.5 per cent had oppositional defiant/conduct disorder.

- Among bully-victims, 21.5 per cent had oppositional defiant/conduct disorder, 17.7 per cent experienced depression and 17.7 per cent had attention-deficit disorder.

- Among victims, 14.4 per cent had attention-deficit disorder, 9.6 per cent experienced depression and 8.7 per cent had anxiety disorder.

- Just over 50 per cent of the children in the study were neither bullies nor victims, and only 23.3 per cent of these had any contact with mental health professionals.

- The rate of contact with professionals was 41 per cent for bullies, 41.7 per cent for bully-victims and 24 per cent for victims.

- Boys were more likely to be bullies and bully-victims than girls; however, boys and girls were victimized equally.

SOURCE

Kumpulainen, K., Kaija, P. & Rasanen, E. (2001). Psychiatric disorders and the use of mental health services among children involved in bullying. *Aggressive Behavior, 27*, 102–110.

Profile of Youth from a Low-Income Urban Community

This paper presents data collected by university researchers from several sources in South Bronx, New York, a low-income urban community. The study was designed to help public health professionals better understand young people's perceptions of violence in the context of their daily lives. The objective was to help young people and communities design effective interventions to reduce violence.

The community:

- Of those aged 15 to 19, over 90 per cent were either Black or Hispanic.

- Households with an annual income of less than $15,000 were 48.2 per cent to 56.3 per cent of the population.

- Homicides per 100,000 were 58.2 per cent to 76.3 per cent of the population compared to 26.7 per cent in New York City as a whole.

Data were collected from:

- a street survey of young people

- a focus group from a public housing project

- a focus group of young women

- three community-based youth intervention programs

- interviews with incarcerated adolescent males.

RESULTS

The street survey of young people

- 23 per cent of the adolescents had been beaten up, 10 per cent stabbed, 8 per cent shot and 89 per cent knew someone who had been beaten up.

- 46 per cent did not feel safe in the building where they lived.

- Young people also described their use of violence or intimidation in the past six months: 61 per cent had pushed, grabbed or shoved someone. The roles of victim and perpetrator were not always easily distinguishable.

- 36 per cent carried a knife, 8 per cent carried a gun in the previous month and 17 per cent had threatened someone with a weapon.

- Alcohol and other drugs were constant in the lives of many young people: 84 per cent had used marijuana and 41 per cent reported binge drinking.
- Young people saw police both as a cause of violence and as protection from violence.

The focus group of young women and the focus group of the public housing project

- In the focus group of young women and the public housing project group, almost everyone had experienced violence recently.
- Young women and men did not report significantly different rates of violent behaviour in the past six months.
- Young women in the focus group explained that they had become more aggressive so they didn't appear weak or afraid.

Interviews with incarcerated adolescent males

- 26 per cent had been physically or sexually abused.
- 11 per cent had attempted suicide sometime in their lives.
- They had been arrested an average of 2.9 times prior to the current arrest.
- Many reported a high level of violence within the correctional facility.
- 40 per cent were in jail on violence-related charges.
- 43 per cent were in jail for drug charges.

IMPLICATIONS

- Youth from this low-income urban neighbourhood saw major influences in their lives such as family, peers, school and neighbourhood as protective factors *and* risk factors. This is unlike youth from high-income groups, who saw most of these factors as protective. Youth from low-income families also felt that other elements in the community, such as gangs, weapons and the police, played both a positive *and* a negative role in their lives. Thus, if violence prevention programs are to succeed, the positive aspects of major and other community influences have to be strengthened.

- Male and female adolescents experience violence differently. Therefore, some programs have to be specially designed for females while others can be designed to suit both genders.

- Youth programs should offer meaningful relationships with caring adults, a safe space to explore options, and opportunities to connect with a wider world.

SOURCE

Freudenberg, N., Roberts, L., Richie, B.E., Taylor, R.T., McGillicuddy, K. & Greene, M.B. (1999). Coming up in the boogie down: The role of violence in the lives of violent adolescents in the South Bronx. *Health Education and Behavior*, 26, 788–805.

Differences between Mothers' and Fathers' Perceptions of Their Children's Antisocial Behaviour

Past studies have shown that how a problem behaviour is seen depends on the nature of the problem and the person perceiving it. It has been shown that

- There is a greater agreement between parents and adolescents about externalized problems (e.g., aggression) than internalized problems (e.g., anxiety, depression). For example, aggressive behaviour is easier to recognize and agree upon than a depressed state of mind.

- Mothers report more problem behaviours in their children than fathers.

- Mothers who are stressed or depressed report more problem behaviours in their children than mothers who are not depressed. Thus, sole reliance on the mother's perception of behaviour problems in their children could lead to inaccurate assessment.

- Fathers seem to be less affected than mothers by their mental state when they perceive problem behaviours in their children.

The present study was designed to see if differences between parents' and adolescents' perception of problem behaviour increases or decreases over a four-year period, and to see if agreement regarding problematic behaviour (or lack of it) depends on the nature of the problem behaviour. Over the course of a four-year longitudinal study, 198 adolescents and their parents participated, completing four surveys (including the Child

Behaviour Checklist and the Youth Self-Report) about externalized and internalized behaviour.

RESULTS

- In all four surveys, male and female adolescents reported more externalized and internalized problem behaviours than their parents.

- Mothers reported more problem behaviours in their children than fathers.

- There was greater agreement between mothers and adolescents than fathers and adolescents in making judgments about the nature of problem behaviours.

- Most parents agreed on the presence of problem behaviour in their children. This did not change as the adolescents aged. This agreement was stronger for externalized behaviours than for internalized behaviours.

- More parents and daughters agreed about problem behaviours than parents and sons.

- Fathers and sons agreed the least for all types of behaviours and agreed the least over time.

- Adolescents, girls in particular, chose their mothers over their fathers to confide in.

- Mothers and fathers both showed greater agreement about their daughters' behaviour than their sons'.

IMPLICATIONS

The information provided by the adolescent is especially important, because parents are not always aware of the adolescent's internal behaviours. Although there is more agreement between adolescents and mothers regarding problem behaviours, mothers experiencing marital discord and depression tend to report more problem behaviours in their children than mothers who are not stressed or depressed.

SOURCE

Seiffge-Krenke, I. & Kollmar, F. (1998). Discrepancies between mothers' and fathers' perceptions of sons' and daughters' problem behaviour: A longitudinal analysis of parent-adolescent agreement on internalizing and externalizing problem behaviour. *Journal of Child Psychology and Psychiatry, 39*, 687–697.

Causes and Contributing Factors

Exposure to Violence and Emotional State

Children in poverty-stricken areas of large cities in the United States are often exposed to violence on a regular basis. A survey of 436 Grade 6 students from three schools in the southeastern United States was conducted from 1994 to 1995. The average age was from 10 to 12 years, and 94 per cent identified themselves as Black or African Americans.

RESULTS

- 91 per cent of girls and 92 per cent of boys had seen someone being beaten up.

- 16 per cent of girls and 37 per cent of boys had been beaten up.

- 30 per cent of girls and 42 per cent of boys had seen someone being shot.

COMMENT

This exposure to violence led to an increase of violent behaviour in girls but not in boys. Because boys reported more exposure to violence and higher initial rates of violent behaviour than girls did, it is possible that they reached a plateau.

This study differs from previous studies in the area of emotional distress. Previous studies suggested that exposure to violence leads to an increase in anxiety, depression and sleep disturbances. The results of the study did not indicate any increase in emotional distress in boys or girls when exposed to violence. It is possible that these children became desensitized to violence, and it stopped affecting their emotional state.

SOURCE

Farrell, A.D. & Bruce, S.E. (1997). Impact of exposure to community violence on violent behavior and emotional distress among urban adolescents. *Journal of Clinical Child Psychology, 26,* 2–14.

Effects on Youth Exposed to Domestic Violence

There is considerable evidence that domestic violence has an impact on child functioning. Children living in families where they are exposed to domestic violence have been shown to be at risk for behavioural, emotional, physical and cognitive difficulties and long-term developmental problems. Furthermore, they have an increased risk of becoming victims of violence themselves (youth crime victimization).

The primary objective of this study was to see how youth are at risk of crime victimization when they live with an adult who has either been the victim of domestic violence or another violent crime. The following three groups were examined:

- youth living in households in which an adult had reported violence by a domestic partner

- youth living in households in which an adult had reported violence by a person not living in the household

- youth living in households in which there had been no victimization reported by any household adult.

RESULTS

- Youth are at a higher risk for crime victimization when they live with a victimized adult.

- Risk increases for youth whether they live with an adult who is victimized by domestic violence or by violence from a non-domestic offender.

- Girls, compared to boys, living in households with an adult victim of domestic violence are at a higher risk for crime victimization.

COMMENT

The results of this study support past research, which has shown that exposure to domestic violence has a negative impact on child functioning. The results extend further and suggest that when an adult experiences violence outside of the home, the impact on the child is similar to witnessing domestic violence. These findings point out the importance of prevention strategies. Children in households where an adult has been victimized in any manner should be given high priority for prevention training and other services that may reduce the risk of future crime victimization.

SOURCE

Mitchell, K.J. & Finkelhor, D. (2001). Risk of crime victimization among youth exposed to domestic violence. *Journal of Interpersonal Violence, 16(9)*, 944–964.

Television and Violent Behaviours

Violent acts are often portrayed on television. In general, children watch three or more hours of TV per day, so they are exposed regularly to violent scenes. Research studies have shown that children who watch a lot of television are at high risk for

• becoming more aggressive

• becoming desensitized to violence occurring in the real world

• developing a perception of the world as a scary and dangerous place.

Thus, there is a relationship between heavy television viewing among children and emotional and behavioural problems.

This study examined how children's television-viewing practices are associated with symptoms of psychological trauma and aggressive behaviours. A total of 2,245 students in grades 2 through 8 completed questions about television-viewing (e.g., hours per day, types of programs preferred), violent behaviours and trauma symptoms they experienced.

RESULTS

• Children who reported watching more than six hours of television per day, compared to those who watched less than five, had significantly higher trauma symptom scores and reported higher levels of violent behaviours.

• Children who reported a preference for shows that contained action and fighting reported higher levels of violent behaviours than children who reported a preference for other types of shows.

• Heavy television viewing was shown to be associated with symptoms of psychological trauma and violent behaviours, but there was no evidence of a causal relationship. Thus, it is possible that children who already have psychological or behavioural problems tend to watch more television than children without such problems. However, it is also possible, and consistent with theory and earlier research, that heavy television-viewing could worsen previously existing emotional and behavioural difficulties.

IMPLICATIONS

The results from this study suggest that parents should monitor the amount of television children watch, particularly violent content. In addition, heavy television viewing may indicate the presence of problems such as depression and anxiety. When psychiatrists and mental health professionals evaluate children, the authors recommend that television-viewing should be explored.

SOURCE

Singer, M.I., Slovak, K., Frierson, T. & York, P. (1998). Viewing preferences, symptoms of psychological trauma and violent behaviors among children who watch television. *Journal of the American Academy of Child and Adolescent Psychiatry*, 37, 1041–1048.

Temperament and Behaviour

The objective of the study was to determine the relationship between behaviour and temperament. Temperament is defined as "genetically determined behavioural and emotional characteristics that a child exhibits during infancy."

In this study, parents of 759 same-sex twins born between 1977 and 1985 were asked to complete the Child Behaviour Checklist to determine behavioural characteristics (i.e., anxiety or depression; attention problems; delinquent or aggressive behaviour). To assess temperamental characteristics (i.e., emotional, sociable, active), parents also completed the EAS Temperament Survey. These questionnaires were sent in 1992 when the twins were between the ages of six and 15. After two years, parents were asked to complete the same questionnaires again as a follow-up.

RESULTS

The children who had a highly emotional temperament:

- cried easily
- got upset easily
- reacted intensely when upset.

Later in life, these highly emotional children were more likely to:

- develop behaviour problems

- experience anxiety and depression

- have difficulty paying attention

- develop delinquent behaviour, such as lying, cheating and stealing (more common in boys)

- develop behaviours such as hitting people and destroying objects (also more common in boys).

Other characteristics of temperament, such as level of activity and sociability, were less influential in determining behaviour. However, a high activity level was related to aggressive behaviour, particularly in young children.

COMMENT

Previous studies have shown that some children are born with a difficult temperament. As babies, these children are hard to feed, are poor sleepers, and are hard to toilet train. These babies are also more likely to grow up with behavioural problems than are babies born with a good temperament, particularly if they grow up in dysfunctional families. Consistent with previous studies, this study suggests that children born with a difficult temperament are more likely to engage in delinquent and aggressive behaviour later in life. However, there is evidence that children with a difficult temperament can grow up to be "normal" in extraordinarily caring and understanding families.

SOURCE

Gjone, H. & Stevenson, J. (1997). A longitudinal twin study of temperament and behavior problems: Common genetic or environmental influences? *Journal of the American Academy of Child and Adolescent Psychiatry, 36*, 1448–1456.

Early Behaviour Problems and Teen Pregnancy

Teenage mothers and their children often deal with many physical, social and emotional problems. To prevent early pregnancy and motherhood, an understanding of the risk factors associated with teen pregnancy is essential. One factor associated with an increased risk of teenage pregnancy is early behavioural problems and difficulties. However, various social and contextual factors, related both to early conduct problems and to teen pregnancy, may account for this association. These factors include:

- social background and disadvantage

- child characteristics

- early parenting and family functioning.

Research has also suggested that children who have early conduct problems are at increased risk, not only for teenage pregnancy and early parenting, but also for a tendency toward increased risk-taking behaviour and norm violation (i.e., early sexual development and behaviour, deviant peer affiliations, early substance use, and disruptive behaviour such as school truancy and difficulties with school authorities).

In this study, the behaviour of a large group of New Zealand girls was studied from infancy to age 18 as part of the Christchurch Health and Development Study (Fergusson et al., 1989).

RESULTS

- The high rate of teenage pregnancy among girls with early behaviour problems reflected their disadvantaged family backgrounds and tendencies toward risk-taking behaviours in adolescence.

- The social/contextual factors found to be significantly related to teenage pregnancy included how much education the mother had, parental changes and mother-daughter interaction that was punitive and happened at an early age. However, the relationship between early behaviour problems and teenage pregnancy was significant even after the social/contextual factors were accounted for. This suggests a possible causal relationship between early behaviour problems and teenage pregnancy.

- The relationship between early behaviour problems and teenage pregnancy appeared to be mediated by a pattern of risk-taking behaviour in adolescence. In other words, girls with early behaviour problems had sexual intercourse at an early age, had multiple sexual partners, used alcohol or drugs and had deviant peer groups or partners.

SOURCE

Woodward, L.J. & Fergusson, D.M. (1999). Early conduct problems and later risk of teenage pregnancy in girls. *Development and Psychopathology, 11,* 127–141.

Fergusson, D.M., Horwood, J.L., Shannon, F.T. & Lawton, J.M. (1989). The Christchurch Child Development Study: A review of epidemiological findings. *Paediatric and Perinatal Epidemiology, 3,* 278–301.

Adult Criminal Behaviour Can Be Predicted

In the Cambridge Study of Delinquent Development, 411 South London males were studied at age eight, interviewed yearly up to age 32, and their criminal records were checked up to age 40. This study reports how psychosocial factors measured at ages eight through 10, and risk scores derived from these, can predict antisocial personality disorder at ages 18 to 32 and criminal convictions between ages 21 and 40. Overall risk scores were determined by adding the number of independent risk factors.

RESULTS

• Males who were convicted as adults tended to have high scores for antisocial behaviour at ages 10, 18 and 32. A number of psychosocial risk factors were found to be independent predictors of these high scores as well as predictors of conviction. For example, having a parent convicted of a crime before the son's 10th birthday was an important explanatory factor in the son's antisocial behaviour at ages 18 and 32, and of being convicted.

• Other important predictors or risk factors included large families, low IQs or attainment, young or nervous mothers, poor child-rearing practices and disrupted families.

• Predictably, the percentage of males who became antisocial and were convicted increased as risk scores grew. For example, at age 18, 67 per cent of males with four or more risk factors out of six became antisocial compared to only 9 per cent of males with none or one of these risk factors present. Similarly, at age 32, 61 per cent of males with three or more risk factors showed antisocial behaviour, compared to only 13 per cent of males with no risk factors. As for convictions, 14 per cent of males with no risk factors were convicted, compared to 64 per cent with three or more risk factors.

COMMENT

Psychosocial risk factors measured at ages eight to 10 can predict antisocial behaviour at ages 18 and 32, and criminal convictions between the ages of 21 and 40, to a surprising degree. Combining different psychosocial risk factors helped identify a very high-risk group at ages eight to 10. Two-thirds of this group became antisocial at age 18 and 60 per cent were antisocial at 32. More research is needed to establish the precise causes linking these risk factors and antisocial behaviour.

SOURCE

Farrington, D.P. (2000). Psychosocial predictors of adult antisocial personality and adult convictions. *Behavioral Sciences & the Law, 18(5)*, 605–622.

Predicting Disruptive Behaviour in Preschoolers

Coercive attachment is the constant struggle between the child and parent/guardian, which leads to distress in the relationship and prevents conflict resolution. Lower levels of marital satisfaction and permissive parenting practices are associated with disruptive behaviour in preschool children.

RESULTS

- Permissive parenting (when a child is non-compliant, and there is a lack of structure, consistency and involvement) can lead to disruptive behaviour in preschool children.

- In preschool children, permissive parenting may play a greater role in the development of disruptive behaviour than authoritarian parenting.

SOURCE

DeVito, C. & Hopkins, J. (2001). Attachment, parenting, and marital dissatisfaction as predictors of disruptive behavior in preschoolers. *Development and Psychopathology, 13(2)*, 215–231.

Predicting Behaviour Problems from Kindergarten Assessments

Childhood aggression is often seen as a good predictor of later antisocial behaviour. The objective of this study was to examine the issue of predicting later problem behaviours from childhood behaviours.

Kindergarten teachers rated the ability of childhood physical aggression, hyperactivity, inattention, anxiety and prosocial behaviour to predict self-reported delinquency, peer-related social withdrawal and school placement in preadolescence.

Person-oriented and variable-oriented approaches were used in this longitudinal study involving 1,034 boys from low socio-economic neighbourhoods. The person-oriented approach is useful when focusing on individuals with particular behaviour patterns. It can be useful in screening those who require preventive interventions. The variable approach has traditionally been used to predict later problem behaviours from childhood behaviours. The variable approach analyses the association between two or more variables, at two or more points in time.

RESULTS

- Both approaches indicated that socio-economic adversity during the preschool years can result in behaviour problems as a child starts school, and can lead to adjustment problems.

- Both approaches indicated that early externalizing problems (e.g., aggressive behaviour) can lead to later externalizing problems such as self-reported delinquency.

- Both approaches indicated that early internalizing problems (e.g., anxiety, depression) can lead to later internalizing problems such as peer-related social withdrawal.

- The person-oriented approach indicated that all patterns of behaviour problems in kindergarten increased the risk for placement in a special class.

- The variable-oriented approach indicated that inattention and a lack of prosocial behaviour increased the risk for placement in a special class.

- The person-oriented approach indicated that kindergarten boys with many problems had the highest percentage of more than one problem during preadolescence.

COMMENT

The findings illustrate that kindergarten teacher ratings of behaviour problems and socio-economic adversity during the preschool years are good predictors of adjustment problems in preadolescence. Preventive or curative interventions should target the active components in the developmental process, which will lead to a given outcome. Gender issues should also be considered for the prediction of future social maladjustment when assessing a child's behaviour patterns.

SOURCE

Haapasalo, J., Tremblay, R.E., Boulerice, B. & Vitaro, F. (2000). Relative advantages of person- and variable-based approaches for predicting problem behaviors from kindergarten assessments. *Journal of Quantitative Criminology, 16(2)*, 145–168.

The Effects of Bullying Behaviours on Primary-School Children

Most studies have focused on behavioural problems associated with direct bullying; however, another kind of bullying has been identified as relational bullying. Relational bullying is described as the hurtful manipulation of peer relationships—inflicting harm on others through behaviours such as social exclusion and malicious rumour-spreading.

This study examined the prevalence of both direct and relational bullying in primary-school children and their relationship to behaviour problems. Individual interviews were conducted with 1,982 children aged six to nine, and 1,639 parents completed a Strengths and Difficulties Questionnaire (SDQ) regarding their children's behaviour.

The goals of this study fall into the following three categories:

1. to investigate, by means of individual interviews, the prevalence of direct and relational bullying among primary school children

2. to examine whether there are differential effects of direct and relational bullying on parent reports of behaviour problems and whether those involved in both forms of bullying show the most behaviour problems

3. to establish the extent of behaviour problems based on parents' reports for children involved in direct or relational bullying as either

- "pure" bullies
- "pure" victims
- bully/victims (children who bully and are victims of bullying)
- children who are not involved in bullying (neutrals).

RESULTS

Direct bullying behaviour:

- 4.3 per cent of children were direct bullies.
- 39.8 per cent of children were victims of direct bullying behaviour.
- 10.2 per cent of children were bullies and victims.

Relational bullying behaviour:

- 1.1 per cent of children were bullies.
- 37.9 per cent of children were victims.
- 5.9 per cent of children were bullies and victims.

COMMENT

The study found that direct bully/victims and children who are involved in both direct and relational bullying had the highest rates of behaviour problems. Children involved in direct bullying had significantly increased total behaviour problems (hyperactivity, conduct problems, peer problem scores and lower prosocial behaviour scores) compared to those not involved in bullying. Children involved in relational bullying who were categorized as bully/victims and victims had similar total behaviour problems but were less pronounced.

The results suggest that children who are involved in bullying and show externalizing and hyperactivity problems at an early stage may be at risk for life-persistent conduct problems. It is possible that different interventions may be needed, depending on the type of problem the child displays.

SOURCE

Wolke, D., Woods, S., Bloomfield, L. & Karstadt, L. (2000). The association between direct and relational bullying and behaviour problems among primary school children. *Journal of Child Psychology and Psychiatry and Allied Disciplines*, 41(8), 989–1002.

Factors Contributing to Bullying

This study was carried out in a large middle school close to a midwestern metropolis, which has a diverse socio-economic population. At midyear, 558 students were given a questionnaire to complete. The study examined the social factors that contribute to the development of bullying during early adolescence: family, adult and peer influences, neighbourhood and school safety concerns, economic status and access to guns.

Bullying is defined as a set of intentional behaviours causing physical and psychological harm to others—including behaviours such as name-calling, teasing, social exclusion and hitting.

RESULTS

- 80.5 per cent of male and female students reported bullying their peers in the past month.

- The use of physical discipline by parents was associated with bullying.

- Those who had friends who indulge in antisocial and illegal activities were more likely to bully.

- Students who were worried about being safe in the neighbourhood and were more exposed to violence were more likely to bully.

- Those who had access to guns were more likely to bully, and surprisingly, 24.2 per cent reported that they can get a gun very easily.

- Students who spent time with adults who were against violent and aggressive behaviour and suggested non-violent ways of dealing with conflict were less likely to indulge in bullying.

- Students who spent more time with adults were less likely to bully.

COMMENT

The following factors affect children's bullying behaviours: parents and their behaviours and attitudes, friends, neighbourhood and exposure to violence. It is suggested that it is more important to see bullying as a behaviour, which occurs in varying degrees in the majority of children, rather than focus on simply identifying the bullies. The study also suggests that school counsellors, in efforts to reduce bullying, should include interventions aimed at parents, peers and social factors including neighbourhoods.

SOURCE

Espelage, D.L., Bosworth, K. & Simon, T.R. (2000). Examining the social context of bullying behaviors in early adolescence. *Journal of Counseling and Development, 78(3),* 326–333.

What Causes Persistent and Severe Antisocial Behaviour?

It has been suggested that youth with antisocial behaviour can be divided into two types: those whose antisocial behaviour tends to last throughout a lifetime (life course persistent (LCP) type), and those who show antisocial behaviour only during adolescence (adolescence limited (AL)).

The LCP type shows persistent, severe and frequent antisocial behaviour across time and situation. It has been suggested that these youth are born with neuropsychological deficiencies that cause problems with reading, writing, listening, problem solving, speech, memory, attention and impulsivity. Child-rearing can be difficult, and if these young people are raised without understanding and support, it can lead to antisocial and aggressive behaviour.

In contrast to youth with LCP antisocial behaviour, youth with AL antisocial behaviour do not have neuropsychological deficiencies. Their displays of antisocial behaviour are attempts to show their autonomy and independence.

This study attempts to test the LCP and AL classifications. The participants in this study were drawn from an ongoing 20-year longitudinal study and included 267 first-born children whose mothers were from high-risk urban populations. These children were studied into adolescence, given a variety of tests and assessed at different ages. The data collected included results from psychological tests, interviews, questionnaires, and observations of interactions between mothers and children.

RESULTS

• The classification that youth who have LCP antisocial behaviour have neuropsychological deficits is unsupported.

• The distinguishable factor between the two groups (LCP and AL) is psychological history.

- Normal development of neuropsychological systems needs a support-ive and growth-promoting environment. Therefore, a child will show neuropsychological deficits as a result of growing up in an adverse environment.

The early-onset/persistent group, which is comparable to the LCP group, was characterized by the following factors:

- likeliness to come from single-family households

- experiences of physical abuse, neglect and inadequate parenting

- mothers who were less sensitive and less supportive.

COMMENT

Temperament and neuropsychological deficits play an important role in explaining persistent and frequent antisocial behaviour. The authors agree that the study has a number of limitations. The sample size is small, and some of the measures of temperament and neuropsychological functioning are not ideal. Most research related to the classification of antisocial youth suggests that persistent and severe antisocial behaviour is associated with difficult temperament and deficits, specifically when children with these deficits are raised in an adverse environment.

SOURCE

Aguilar, B., Sroufe, A.L., Egeland, B. & Carlson, E. (2000). Distinguishing the early-onset/persistent and adolescent-onset antisocial behavior types: From birth to 16 years. *Development and Psychopathology*, *12*, 109–132.

Impulsivity and Antisocial Behaviour

Although impulsivity is a symptom of many psychiatric disorders, it is seldom clearly defined. Impulsivity plays a key role in conduct disorder and attention-deficit disorder, but it is seldom measured and treated.

Definition

Impulsivity is defined as a predisposition to rapid, unplanned reactions to internal or external stimuli and a disregard for the negative consequences of these reactions (which can affect the individual and others). Impul-sivity is defined as a predisposition—part of a pattern of behaviour rather than a single act. This distinction is important to clinicians, because peo-ple with impulsive aggression react differently to medications than people with premeditated aggression.

Measuring impulsivity

- Self-report measures, including the Barratt Impulsiveness Scale and Eysenck Impulsiveness Questionnaire, are good ways to determine the presence of impulsivity and its intensity.

- Behavioural laboratory measures include punishment and/or extinction (ignoring behaviour to avoid reinforcing it) types of measures. The advantage of these measures is that they are suitable for repeated use.

- Event-related potential involves recording brain activity while a person performs various tasks.

Impulsivity in psychiatric disorders

Impulsivity plays a significant role in the following disorders:

- antisocial personality disorder
- borderline personality disorder
- substance abuse/dependence
- bipolar disorder
- attention-deficit hyperactivity disorder
- conduct disorder.

Treatment of impulsivity

The following approaches have been used with some success:

- Cognitive behaviour psychotherapy involves training in interpersonal problem-solving skills. It has been successful in reducing impulsivity in children.

- Contingency management involves the use of predetermined positive or negative consequences to reward or punish a target behaviour.

- Pharmacological treatment includes the use of drugs such as methylphenidate (Ritalin), risperidone and lithium.

COMMENT

Research has been limited in this area, as impulsivity has been seen as a symptom of various disorders rather than a problem in itself. In the past, the classification of conduct disorder included two types: unsocialized and socialized, which were distinguished primarily by the presence or absence of impulsivity. The unsocialized group was said to be aggressive or impulsive, while the socialized group premeditated aggressive behaviour. Some clinicians think this differentiation had value, as the unsocialized group was said to respond to medication while the socialized group did not. This distinction does not exist in the DSM-IV.

SOURCE

Moeller, F.G., Barratt, E.S., Dougherty, D.M, Schmitz, J.M & Swann, A.C. (2001). Psychiatric aspects of impulsivity. *American Journal of Psychiatry, 158(11)*, 1783–1793.

Reading Disability and Problem Behaviours

This study investigated the association between reading problems and symptoms of anxiety, depression and disruptive behaviour. The sample was taken from twins aged eight to 18, attending public schools from 27 school districts within 150 miles of Denver and Boulder, Colorado. If one of the twins from a pair had a reading difficulty based on a history of reading problems and met the reading achievement cut-off score, he or she was identified as having a reading problem. In pairs of twins in which one but not the other had a reading problem, both twins were included in the study; in pairs in which both had the disability, one twin was included in the study.

To assess child psychopathology, parents were interviewed and also asked to complete behaviour-rating scales about their children. The children were also interviewed and asked to complete a self-report of symptoms of depression.

RESULTS

- Children with reading difficulties had significantly lower IQs and socio-economic status than children without reading difficulties.

- Children with reading difficulties showed significantly more emotional and disruptive behavioural problems even when effects of IQ and socio-economic status were accounted for.

- Boys with reading difficulties were more likely than girls to have ADHD and aggressive behaviour.

- Girls with reading difficulties were more likely to have depression than boys, and had various somatic complaints, such as headaches and stomach aches because of stress.

- In boys and girls both, attention-deficit hyperactivity disorder was the category that was most often associated with reading problems.

COMMENT

Although past studies have associated reading disability with aggressive behaviour, this is the first study associating reading disability, depression and somatic symptoms.

SOURCE

Willcutt, E.G. & Pennington, B.F. (2000). Psychiatric comorbidity in children and adolescents with reading disability. *Journal of Child Psychology and Psychiatry and Allied Disciplines, 41(8)*, 1039–1048.

Parenting and Hyperactivity

This study showed that parents of hyperactive children, compared to parents of a control group, showed:

- poor coping skills
- aggressive discipline
- feelings of hostility and anger.

RESULTS

- It is easier for the parents of children in the control group (who are better behaved) to parent effectively because they are more able to identify problems and predict solutions in advance, thus avoiding conflict.
- On the other hand, it is possible that because parents of hyperactive children are less effective in child management, they contribute to conflicts that could have been avoided.

COMMENT

This study does not suggest that hyperactivity is caused by parental behaviour. However, it challenges the commonly held view that psychosocial factors only play a minor role in understanding and treating hyperactivity. Parental behaviour and other social factors should be more closely examined, as they play a significant role in the treatment, course and prognosis of hyperactivity.

SOURCE

Woodward, L., Taylor, E. & Dowdney, L. (1998). The parenting and family functioning of children with hyperactivity. *Journal of Child Psychology and Psychiatry*, 39, 161–169.

Fathers and Preschool Behaviour Problems

Although most studies tend to focus on the characteristics of mothers of children with behaviour problems, this study focused on the fathers' characteristics.

Compared to fathers of preschool children who had not been referred to a child psychiatry clinic, fathers of preschool children who had been referred reported:

- more frequent use of harsh punishment

- more stressful life events

- more psychological symptoms

- less satisfaction with their parenting roles

- less positive involvement with their children.

RESULTS

- A father's use of harsh punishment may be the most useful characteristic in identifying which preschoolers will be referred to a clinic.

- It is important to include fathers in a child's assessment and treatment.

SOURCE

DeKlyen, M., Biernbaum, M.A., Speltz, M.L. & Greenberg, M.T. (1998). Fathers and Preschool Behaviour Problems. *Developmental Psychology*, 34, 264–275.

Absentee Fathers: Impact on Antisocial Behaviour in Families

This study examined whether the presence or absence of biological fathers was associated with increased antisocial behaviour in families. The problem with many studies that target fathers of antisocial children is that many of the fathers are not available for participation or cannot even be located. Father departure rates range from 20 per cent to as high as 75 per cent in these families.

Investigators studied relationships between antisocial behaviour and three paternal conditions:

- two-parent families
- separated but recruitable fathers
- fathers who refused to participate or could not be located.

The antisocial symptoms were collected for 161 clinic-referred children and their parents.

RESULTS

- Families with fathers at home had fewer paternal, maternal and child antisocial symptoms, and scored higher on multiple socio-economic status (SES) indicators, than families with departed fathers did.
- Antisocial characteristics were highest and SES indicators lowest when fathers could not be located or recruited.
- Antisocial behaviour in any family member was more likely if the father did not participate.
- The heightened antisocial behaviour in children associated with absent biological fathers was not changed by the presence of stepfathers nor was it accounted for by lower SES.

Hypotheses were advanced to explain these results:

- Father departure deprives the family in a number of ways (diminished father relationship, disrupted family structure, reduced supervision, etc.). These deprivations cause children to become more antisocial. Therefore, if the biological father leaves, restoring a father figure might help child behaviour problems. However, in the families separated from biological fathers, child antisocial behaviour did not significantly differ between those with and without a stepfather.
- A common genetic factor might explain both father departure and increased child antisocial behaviour: (1) Increasing degrees of anti-social personality in fathers are reflected in more separation and diminished contact with the family. (2) Antisocial personality is partly genetic and can run in families. Therefore child antisocial behaviour can be related to parental antisocial behaviour, whether the biological father is part of the family or not.

COMMENT

The relationship between paternal antisocial personality disorder (APD) and child conduct disorder (CD) is well documented. Psychopathy has been associated with an inherited structural abnormality in the frontal lobes and/or a chemical imbalance of the brain.

Adoption studies and studies of twins confirm a genetic link, though this can change in a positive environment. Father departure or disappearance is not a random event; people with APD are less likely to sustain intimate partnerships and acknowledge family responsibilities.

It is noteworthy that this study showed that the presence of stepfathers did not affect the likelihood of antisocial behaviour in the child. After a biological father departed, the introduction of a stepfather raised the family's income but did not improve the child's behaviour.

If positive child socialization is to be successful, specialized parenting strategies and professional guidance may therefore be needed, not only for the single mothers of problem children whose partners have departed, but also for the stepfathers who join these families.

SOURCE

Pfiffner, L.J., McBurnett, K., Rathouz, P.J. (2001). Father absence and familial antisocial characteristics. *Journal of Abnormal Child Psychology, 29(5)*, 357–367.

Effects of Family and Friends on Antisocial Behaviour in Youth

In this study, youth whose criminal offenses were chronic and severe were randomly assigned to two different conditions; 23 were assigned to residential group care and 30 were assigned to multi-dimensional-treatment foster care (MTFC).

Group care involved six to 15 youth living in a group home where the staff rotated shifts. Most group homes used a positive-peer-culture approach where youths were encouraged to support each other. The youths received individual and group therapy, and ongoing contact with family members was encouraged.

MTFC involved finding foster parents who had experience with adolescents. Each couple was given 20 hours of training before a teenager was placed with them. Training focused on the use of behaviour management to help establish and maintain a structured, individualized living environment. In addition, the teens received individual and family therapy with their natural family, and home visits were used to practice their skills in the context of the family milieu.

RESULTS

When treatment ended a year later, the MTFC group differed significantly from the group care, moving in a positive direction on all measured variables:

- lower antisocial behaviour
- better scores in family management
- lower deviant-peer association scores.

COMMENT

The study's results support the ideas that

- Exposing youth to other delinquent peers is risky.
- Providing an environment with firm limits and positive interaction between youths and caretakers is beneficial.

SOURCE

Eddy, J.M. & Chamberlain, P. (2000). Family management and deviant peer association as mediators of the impact of treatment condition on youth antisocial behavior. *Journal of Consulting and Clinical Psychology, 68(5),* 857–863.

Peer Relationships and Antisocial Behaviour

These studies asked the controversial question: How much influence do deviant peers have in determining the antisocial behaviour of youth? From the evidence presented below, the influence of deviant peers becomes critical only when the adolescents have behaviour problems in childhood and when they lack a close, warm and confiding relationship with their parents.

Childhood predictors of deviant peer relationships

Study 1

This study examined children who were having problems with their peers when they were nine years old and studied their behaviour up to the age of 18. The objectives of the study were to determine:

- how these children would behave psychosocially at age 18

- the extent to which peer relationship problems caused difficult and antisocial behaviour later on

- whether peer problems at age nine were related to social background and quality of the child-parent relationship.

A large group of girls from New Zealand were studied extensively from birth as part of the Christchurch Health and Developmental Study (CHDS). Teachers were asked to rate the quality of children's peer relationships at age nine. At 18, participants completed questionnaires examining a range of psychosocial outcomes.

RESULTS

- By age 18, children with high rates of early peer-relationship problems were at increased risk of externalizing behaviour problems such as criminal offending and problem substance use.

- Child and family factors associated both with early peer-relationship problems and with adjustment later on largely explained the above association.

- Contrary to several other studies, no association was found between children's peer functioning and later risks of anxiety disorder or major depression.

- The extent of children's early conduct problems was the most important factor in explaining associations between peer-relationship problems and adjustment later in life.

COMMENT

While an association was found between early peer-relationship problems and increased risk of behaviour problems, this relationship was not causal. Rather, the most influential variable was the measure of childhood conduct problems (e.g., aggression and cruelty to others, destruction of property, temper outbursts, tendencies to interpret ambiguous behavioural cues of other children as hostile provocations, lying, stealing, etc.). Therefore, the socially difficult behaviours of children with early conduct problems may account for these children's poor peer acceptance and the apparent associations found between childhood peer relations and adjustment later on.

SOURCE

Woodward, L.J. & Fergusson, D.M. (1999). Childhood peer relationship problems and psychosocial adjustment in late adolescence. *Journal of Abnormal Child Psychology, 27,* 87–104.

Study 2

RESULTS

Results were gathered over the course of the CHDS:

- Adolescent peer affiliations were associated with a wide range of prospectively measured social, family, parental and individual factors. This analysis indicated that those children most at risk of forming deviant peer affiliations were those from socially disadvantaged backgrounds and/or dysfunctional families. The children also had early-onset conduct problems and other difficulties.

- Increased risks of deviant later peer relations were associated with:

  - low family socio-economic status

  - parental conflict

  - poor mother and child interaction

  - childhood sexual abuse

  - parental alcoholism, criminal offending, illicit drug use or smoking

  - early conduct problems

  - early anxiety or withdrawal

  - early smoking experimentation.

COMMENT

The authors concluded that peer affiliations in adolescence are shaped by complex social, family and individual processes that include social stratification, family functioning and individual behavioural predispositions.

SOURCE

Fergusson, D.M. & Horwood, L.J. (1999). Prospective childhood predictors of deviant peer affiliations in adolescence. *Journal of Child Psychology and Psychiatry, 40*, 581–592.

Deviant peers and disruptive behaviour

Study 3

In this study, three developmental models were tested using a program designed to prevent disruptive behaviour. The intervention program was implemented over a two-year period for children aged seven to nine. Participants were 73 boys who were judged by their teachers as disruptive; 34 of them formed a control group.

The program included training in alternative, appropriate social and problem-solving skills to reduce disruptive behaviour. It was believed that by becoming less disruptive, these children would be accepted by less deviant peers. In addition, parents were taught skills (e.g., use of reinforcement contingencies and sustained supervision) to reduce disruptive behaviour in the home and to help boys select less deviant peers.

The following three models for the development of conduct problems were tested:

1. The peer influence model: deviant friends play a causal role, which later leads to conduct disorder or delinquency. According to this model, if we facilitate non-deviant peer association during early adolescence, later conduct problems will be positively affected.

2. The individual characteristics model: childhood disruptive behaviours independently lead to antisocial behaviour and to incidental association with deviant peers. According to this model, if we reduce early disruptiveness, it will have a direct impact on later conduct problems.

3. An interaction of peer influence characteristics and individual characteristics: association with deviant peers and disruptive behaviours interact in some way, leading to later conduct problems.

RESULTS

• The results of the study supported the third hypothesis that, while associating with less deviant friends had a positive effect, the outcome depended on whether the disruptive behaviour of the child had been reduced by participating in the program.

SOURCE

Vitaro, F., Brendgen, M., Pagani, L., Tremblay, R.E. & McDuff, P. (1999). Disruptive behavior, peer association, and conduct disorder. Testing the developmental links through early intervention. *Development and Psychopathology*, 11, 287–304.

Adolescent problem behaviour: The influence of parents and peers

Study 4

This was a two-year study of 204 adolescents and parents who completed a series of self-report questionnaires.

RESULTS

- Families having high levels of conflict were more likely to have low levels of parent-child involvement.

- High levels of family conflict were related to poor parental monitoring and association with deviant peers one year later.

- At a two-year follow-up, poor parental monitoring and associations with deviant peers were strong predictors of an array of problem behaviours, including:

  - antisocial behaviour

  - high-risk sex

  - academic failure

  - substance use.

- For a large number of adolescents, the above problem behaviours were interrelated.

- Despite evidence of increasing peer influence among adolescents, parents can continue to be a source of influence throughout adolescence.

COMMENT

For intervention, the authors suggest an integrated prevention effort that strengthens parenting practices, monitors norms in the community and provides social skills early in the developmental process. These efforts will provide a powerful and cost-effective set of prevention procedures.

SOURCE

Ary, D.V., Duncan, T.E., Duncan, S.C. & Hops, H. (1999). Adolescent problem behavior: The influence of parents and peers. *Behaviour Research and Therapy, 37*, 217–230.

Peer Group Victimization

There is some evidence that a small group of children in schools are persistently targeted for physical and verbal abuse by other children. This study was designed to assess the effect of such abuse on the children's behaviour and development. A group of 330 children in grades 3 or 4 were assessed for aggression, victimization and rejection by peers. After a period of two years, these children were assessed again for behaviour problems. This assessment was completed by parents and teachers using standardized behaviour checklists.

RESULTS

- Children who are often bullied by their peers are likely to develop behaviour problems in school and at home.

- These problems are more likely to be externalized (aggression-related) and attention-related than internalized (anxiety- and depression-related).

COMMENT

It is evident that children who experience bullying are affected. Past studies suggest that children who are bullied are more likely to become withdrawn and submissive than aggressive. However, they may react by becoming aggressive or depressed and withdrawn.

SOURCE

Schwartz, D., McFadyen-Ketchum, S.A., Dodge, K.A., Pettit, G.S. & Bates, J.E. (1998). Peer group victimization as a predictor of children's behavior problems at home and in school. *Development and Psychopathology, 10*, 87–99.

Prevention

Predicting Antisocial Behaviour in Children

Past studies have shown that:

- Behaviour problems are present in very young children, and these problems remain stable over a number of years.

- Stable externalizing problems (e.g., aggressive behaviour) are stronger than internalizing problems (e.g., anxiety, depression).

- The primary reason for the development of antisocial behaviour in a child is poor child management practices in the family.

- Improper discipline in early childhood leads to coercive interactions between the child and the parents. As a result, the child learns antisocial behaviours rather than prosocial behaviours.

In this study, 156 children at 18 months of age were observed in playgroups to determine if observations would match teachers' ratings of externalizing behaviour at age five.

RESULTS

The following factors at 18 months were found to be predictors of later externalizing behaviour at age five:

- negative behaviour in the toddler playgroup (as rated by the teacher)

- parents' negative and inappropriate behaviour toward the child at home

- single-mother family status.

COMMENT

Children under six who show difficult behaviour in playgroups can be identified, and their parents can be given help. This may prevent aggressive and non-compliant behaviour when the children enter school.

SOURCE

Fagot, B.I. & Leve, L.D. (1998). Teacher ratings of externalizing behaviour at school entry for boys and girls: Similar early predictors and different correlates. *Journal of Child Psychology and Psychiatry, 39*, 555–566.

Identifying High-Risk Children

Study 1

Children with disruptive, non-compliant and externalizing behaviour (e.g., aggression, hyperactivity) are at high risk for developing antisocial behaviour later in life. Interventions that target these children at an early age would therefore be most effective because they catch the behaviour before it escalates and at a time when change is easier. So we know it is important to identify high-risk children early to prevent further antisocial behaviour, but how can we make sure that these children are properly identified?

Research has suggested that children as young as four or five with troublesome externalizing behaviours have a 50 per cent or greater chance of developing persistent behaviour problems. However, very few well-designed studies have addressed how accurately early externalizing behaviour problems can predict future behaviour problems in non-clinic populations. In addition, other characteristics about the child that may be useful predictors (i.e., socio-economic disadvantages, maternal depression, poor parenting practices) have not been addressed in many studies.

This study examines the predictive accuracy of externalizing behaviour separately and in combination with other child and familial risk factors. Non-clinic populations of children in kindergarten and Grade 1 were studied over a 30-month period.

RESULTS

- When only externalizing symptoms are used to predict behaviour problems in non-clinic populations, many children are likely to be misclassified.

- When other risk factors are evaluated in addition to externalizing symptoms, there is some gain in predictive accuracy.

- There are two disadvantages of misclassifying children at risk:

  - Some children who need help will not be identified as high risk and therefore will remain unserved.

  - On the other hand, some children who have little or no need for intervention will receive treatment unnecessarily, and therefore, will be subject to the risks associated with stigma.

COMMENT

Despite these findings, the authors maintain that targeted interventions may still offer advantages. Many more children will be reached through programs targeted at non-clinic populations than through clinical services alone.

In addition, compared with universal programs, targeted programs are a more efficient way to use resources. There is no doubt that children benefit from early intervention; we just need to find more accurate ways of identifying these children.

SOURCE

Bennett, K.J., Brown, S., Lipman, E.L., Racine, Y., Boyle, M.H. & Offord, D.R. (1999). Predicting conduct problems: Can high-risk children be identified in kindergarten and Grade 1? *Journal of Consulting and Clinical Psychology, 67*, 470–480.

Study 2

This study looked at the effectiveness of two simple questionnaires:

1. Inattention/Overactivity with Aggression (IOWA): Conners brief rating scale for teachers. The scale consists of 10 behavioural descriptive items, five related to inattention and overactivity and five related to aggression. Each item is rated from "not at all" to "very much" with answers scored from zero to three.

2. Conners Abbreviated Symptom Questionnaire (CASQ): This questionnaire is completed by parents, and the items tap into observable behaviours related to inattention, overactivity and impulsivity. There are 10 items and they are scored the same way as IOWA.

RESULTS

- By using the two questionnaires, it is possible to identify children with disruptive behaviour problems (i.e., inattention, aggression and non-compliance) with reasonable certainty.

- These two instruments could serve as an initial strategy for screening children in the school setting.

SOURCE

Casat, C.D., Norton, H.J. & Boyle-Whitesel, M. (1999). Identification of elementary school children at risk for disruptive behavioral disturbance: Validation of a combined screening method. *Journal of the American Academy of Child and Adolescent Psychiatry, 38,* 1246–1253.

Infant Temperament and Early Intervention: A 15-Year Follow-Up Study

It has been recognized that some infants are born with a good temperament and some with a difficult temperament. There are various definitions of temperament. In this study, temperament includes two components: (1) fussiness and crying, and (2) demanding behaviour (the need for constant attention due to the inability to entertain oneself).

There have been questions about the relationship between difficult temperament and the development of psychiatric symptoms in adolescence. It has been suggested that difficult temperament alone is unlikely to predict behaviour problems later in life. However, difficult temperament when combined with dysfunctional parental behaviour can lead to clinical disorders in adolescence.

In this study, mothers were asked to complete the Carey Infant Temperament Questionnaire when children were six months old. Parents were also counselled by qualified psychiatric nurses, who visited the families every four to six weeks. The counsellors were supervised weekly by child psychiatrists. The home visits continued until the children were five years old.

When the children were 14 or 15, their psychiatric symptoms were assessed using the Child Behaviour Checklist and the Youth Self-Report. The study was based on the complete data from 100 children (the data was collected in infancy and in adolescence). Fifty-four children received family counselling during the first five years of their lives (10 times per year), and 46 children served as a control group for counselling.

RESULTS

- A fussy or demanding temperament in infancy can predict psychiatric symptoms in adolescence.

- A family counselling program administered during infancy protected the children from developing psychiatric symptoms in adolescence. It allowed the parents to identify the profile of their child's temperament, accept it and to modify their expectations, therefore having a "goodness of fit."

- It may be possible to improve the psychosocial prognosis of children at temperamental risk by home-based intervention focused on parent-child interaction.

SOURCE

Teerikangas, O.M., Aronen, E.T., Martin, R.P. & Huttunen, M.O. (1998). Effects of infant temperament and early intervention on the psychiatric symptoms of adolescents. *Journal of the American Academy of Child and Adolescent Psychiatry, 37*, 1070–1076.

Preventing the Development of Antisocial Behaviour

Considerable evidence suggests that prevention is more cost-effective than treating antisocial behaviour after it has become an established pattern.

In this study, 678 Grade 1 children in nine Baltimore City public schools were randomly assigned to three conditions:

- classroom-centered intervention
- family-school partnership intervention
- control group that received no intervention.

Classroom-centred intervention (CC)

The three components of this intervention included curriculum enhancement, improved-behaviour management practices and backup strategies for children who failed to respond adequately to the intervention.

Family-school partnership intervention (FSP)

This intervention was designed to improve achievement and reduce early aggressive behaviour, shy behaviour and concentration problems. It enhanced parent-teacher communication and gave parents effective teaching and child-behaviour management strategies.

After pre-test assessment in the early fall, the interventions were administered over the Grade 1 year. The impact of the intervention was assessed in the spring of the grades one and two.

RESULTS

- Children who underwent the CC and FSP interventions did better in math and reading than did children in the control group. The largest improvement was seen in children who were doing poorly before the intervention.

- Children who received the CC intervention demonstrated significantly fewer behaviour problems, as rated by teachers, at the end of both first and second grade. For children who received the FSP intervention, behaviour also improved by the end of first grade, but the improvement did not reach a statistically significant level until the follow-up at the end of the second grade.

- In the spring of first grade, a significant number of peers nominated fewer boys as aggressive in the CC group than boys in the control group. No significant effects were found for CC girls or FSP girls or boys. (Although fewer boys in the FSP group were nominated by peers as aggressive compared to the control group, the difference was not statistically significant.)

COMMENT

This is yet another study showing that early intervention can reduce aggressive behaviour and improve academic achievement. Although the follow-up in this study was under two years, many studies show that the results of early intervention last through adolescence and adulthood.

SOURCE

Ialongo, N.S., Werthamer, L., Kellam, S.G., Brown, C.H., Wang, S. & Lin, Y. (1999). Proximal impact of two first-grade preventive interventions on the early risk behaviors for later substance abuse, depression, and antisocial behavior. *American Journal of Community Psychology, 27,* 599–641.

Is Increased Income a Protective Factor against Violence?

This U.S. study examined the association of household income, race/ethnicity and exposure to violence in a nationally representative sample of youth aged 12 to 17.

The youth were classified into three income groups: lower, middle and upper and into three racial groups: Caucasian, African-American and

Hispanic. The youth completed a telephone interview that assessed lifetime occurrences of witnessing violence and receiving physically abusive punishment, physical assault and sexual assault. It was predicted that rates of each type of victimization would decrease as household income increased.

RESULTS

- As household incomes increased, rates for all types of violence decreased for Caucasian youth but not African-American or Hispanic youth.

- In lower-income households, rates of physically abusive punishment were similar. However in the upper-income group, African-American youth reported significantly higher rates (16.8 per cent) compared to Caucasian (6.1 per cent) and Hispanic (5.9 per cent) youth.

- The reported rate for physical assault on African-American youth from upper-income households was 25.6 per cent, nearly twice that of Caucasian youth.

- At the upper-income level, African-American youth also reported significantly higher rates of sexual assault at 15.2 per cent, compared to 7.1 per cent for Hispanics and 4.6 per cent for Caucasians.

COMMENT

This study reveals that protective effects associated with higher-income households are absent for minority groups.

Violence prevention efforts that focus on lower-income families may exclude African-American and Hispanic youth from higher-income households, who may be as much at risk as their lower-income counterparts. One should also consider that many minority families change their income level within one generation, and that parental behaviour may be determined by the lower-income environment that the parent was exposed to during childhood.

SOURCE

Crouch, J.L., Hanson, R.F., Saunders, B.E., Kilpatrick, D.G. & Resnick, H.S. (2000). Income, race/ethnicity and exposure to violence in youth: Results from the national survey of adolescents. *Journal of Community Psychology, 28(6)*, 625–641.

Visiting Mothers during and after Pregnancy Helps

This paper describes a program of research in which nurses visited first time mothers-to-be who were unmarried, adolescent or poor, or a combination of these. This program was developed with the belief that many intractable problems faced by the parents and children are related to

- maternal health-related behaviours during pregnancy (e.g., use of alcohol, tobacco and illegal drugs)
- inadequate care of the children, which leads to neglect, abuse and accidental childhood injuries, which in turn can lead to antisocial and violent behaviour as the child grows up.

During the second trimester of pregnancy, mothers-to-be were visited once a week by a nurse, who had formal training in women's and children's health and competence in managing complex clinical situations. For the rest of the pregnancy, nurses visited the mothers every other week until the birth of the baby. The nurse visited weekly for six weeks after the baby was born, and twice a month from the second to 21st postnatal month. From the 21st to 24th postnatal month, the visits were once a month. (Follow-up assessments were conducted when the children were 15.)

The visits lasted 75 to 90 minutes and were aimed at:

- promoting improvement in women's behaviours, as poor behaviours may adversely affect pregnancy outcome
- helping women build supportive relationships with family and friends
- linking women and their family members to other needed health and human services.

RESULTS

- The program benefited the neediest families (e.g., low-income unmarried women), but provided little benefit to the broader population.
- The rates of childhood injuries, abuse and neglect were reduced.
- Mothers were encouraged to defer future pregnancies. They were helped to find work and become economically self-sufficient, which in turn helped them and their children.

- When the youths were followed up on at 15 years of age, it was dis-
  covered that nurse visitations had a positive effect for them also. These
  children had fewer arrests and convictions, smoked and drank less and
  had fewer sexual partners.

SOURCE

Olds, D.L., Henderson Jr., C.R., Kitzman, H.J., Eckenrode, J.J., Cole, R.E. &
Tatelbaum, R.C. (1999). Prenatal and infancy home visitation by nurses:
Recent findings. *The Future of Children*, *9*, 44–65.

Neighbourhood Solutions for Neighbourhood Problems

Most interventions aimed at antisocial and violent behaviour in youth are
designed and carried out by agencies. This paper describes an intervention that was designed and carried out within a neighbourhood.

A neighbourhood intervention is preferred to an agency intervention for
two reasons: First, several neighbourhood characteristics (e.g., availability of drugs, adult crime, exposure of children to crime) influence the
development of antisocial behaviour in youth. Second, most financial
resources are spent on programs for youth from high-crime areas who are
placed in treatment facilities away from home. Thus, these programs do
not have an impact on the neighbourhood to which the children will
eventually return. Such out-of-home placements have been found to be
ineffective and expensive. As the results of this neighbourhood intervention are not yet available, the paper focuses on the development and
process of intervention.

The project was the result of a collaboration between a university research
centre and neighbourhood stakeholders. The aim was to address key pri-
orities in the neighbourhood and to promote family and neighbourhood
contexts conducive to prosocial youth behaviour.

Selecting a neighbourhood

The first step was to identify potential sites with high levels of youth violence. Eight sites with high rates of poverty, unemployment, child maltreatment, arrests and school problems were identified. One U.S. site,
Union Heights, was selected at random, and other sites were selected to
serve as control groups.

Forming a partnership with neighbourhood stakeholders

Union Heights' representatives were told that the university centre wanted to form a collaborative partnership. The representatives were asked to decide which child and family problems they wanted to address. They were told about the philosophy of the centre and that all interventions would require family and neighbourhood collaboration.

Prioritizing problems affecting youths and families

The top six youth antisocial behaviour problems identified by the representatives were violent crime, substance abuse, drug dealing, child prostitution, vandalism and school expulsions.

Designing and implementing interventions

For youth clinical needs, the multi-systemic approach was chosen as the type of intervention.

For youths at risk of suspension or expulsion, a points system was used. Students would be flagged as being in danger of suspension when they lost a certain number of points for behaviour problems. Teachers would get extra help, provided by the advocacy group (with representatives from the university centre and community) to keep the youth in school.

To accommodate after-school and summer vacation activities for youth, prosocial, recreational, educational and vocational programs were implemented.

COMMENT

Involving not only the family but also the neighbourhood in dealing with antisocial and violent youth is a novel approach that seems promising; however, the results of this intervention have yet to be published. When the results of this study are published, we will have a better idea of the strategy's effectiveness and the value of the enormous effort involved in this type of approach.

SOURCE

Randall, J., Swenson, C.C. & Henggeler, S.W. (1999). Neighborhood solutions for neighborhood problems: An empirically based violence prevention collaboration. *Health Education and Behavior, 26,* 806–820.

Preventing Antisocial Behaviour in Schools

This article reports on the development and testing of a comprehensive model intervention, called First Step to Success, to detect and remedy antisocial behaviour patterns at the point of school entry.

First Step to Success program

First Step to Success is:

- a combined home and school intervention that also contains universal screening procedures to identify children in kindergarten who show signs of antisocial behaviour

- an intervention that targets the three groups of people who have the greatest influence on the developing child (i.e., parents or caregivers, teachers and peers)

- aimed at preventing children in kindergarten from carrying on with antisocial patterns of behaviour, and at the same time, teaching them the skills they need to build effective, teacher- and peer-related skills, and social and behavioural skills.

The First Step to Success program was carried out and evaluated over a two-year period. Two groups of children (a total of 46) in kindergarten were identified as being at-risk and were exposed to the program. Children were randomly assigned to either the experimental or wait-list control group (who participated in the program one year later). Results from the two groups were used to evaluate the intervention's effects and to establish a causal relationship between the intervention and the documented changes in child behaviour.

After completing the program, each target student scored within the normative range on the two most important measures used to evaluate the program. The first measure was the aggression subscale of the Child Behaviour Checklist (CBCL). The second measure was the academic engaged time (AET), which measures the time spent attending to teacher-led activities. This is an important correlate of academic performance and provides a sensitive and reliable measure of behaviour change in the classroom.

RESULTS

- The paper concludes that "mounting universal screening procedures to detect emerging antisocial behaviour patterns among kindergarten and primary grade-level programs represents one of the best options available for reducing the rising tide of antisocial behaviour in schools."

- The authors explain why the intervention is important: "Powerful evidence suggests that antisocial children and youth follow a developmental trajectory in which the antisocial acts they engage in become more serious. Their early identification and exposure to interventions designed to divert them from this path is clearly in the public interest. As public policy, this strategy could save millions of dollars in later incarceration costs."

SOURCE

Walker, H.M., Kavanagh, K., Stiller, B., Golly, A., Severson, H.H. & Feil, E.G. (1998). First step to success: An early intervention approach for preventing school antisocial behavior. *Journal of Emotional and Behavioral Disorders, 6*, 66–80.

Preventing Drug Use in Schools

Reviews of drug prevention programs show that the most promising approaches target people during the beginning of adolescence and teach drug resistance skills in combination with general personal and social skills.

Effective resistance training has three social influence components:

- teaching students to recognize high-risk situations (including peer pressure)

- increasing awareness of pro-drug media influences (movies, TV, rock videos, music, etc.)

- refusal skills training (form, content and rehearsal of effective refusal responses).

An adolescent's pro-drug thoughts, attitudes and beliefs influence drug use. These factors in combination with poor personal and social skills are believed to increase susceptibility to drug use.

Drug prevention programs, which include generic self-management and social skills training (or life skills training), have shown initial smoking prevention effects of 40 per cent to 80 per cent. Booster sessions have enhanced outcomes to 87 per cent.

One large long-term study measured the effects of 15 drug prevention sessions in Grade 7, 10 booster sessions in Grade 8 and five booster sessions in Grade 9. No intervention took place during grades 10 through 12.

RESULTS

At the end of Grade 12, rates of smoking, alcohol and marijuana use were 44 per cent lower for trainees versus non-participants. Prevention effects extended to illicit drug use and lasted a reasonable amount of time after high school.

SOURCE

Botvin, G.J. (2000). Preventing drug abuse in schools: Social and competence enhancement approaches targeting individual-level etiologic factors. *Addictive Behaviors, 25(6)*, 887–897.

School-Based Prevention Programs

Behavioural problems, including criminal activities and substance use, are common in adolescence, and many youth who engage in serious criminal behaviour also use alcohol and other drugs. The co-occurrence of behaviours such as aggression, truancy, poor school achievement, suspensions and drug use during high school is of serious concern because these behaviours are harmful and costly to society.

Recent reviews of programs to prevent substance use prevention and programs to reduce conduct problems and delinquent behaviour have, in general, concluded that at least some forms of these approaches are effective at reducing problem behaviours. However, beyond the fact that something works, there is little understanding about the magnitude of these effects or the characteristics of effective programs.

This study examined effective school-based prevention programs to determine how they prevent or reduce crime, substance use, truancy and other conduct problems. This study summarized, using meta-analytic techniques, results from 165 studies of various prevention programs based in the school system or programs administered by school staff.

RESULTS

- School-based prevention programs appear useful for reducing alcohol and drug use, truancy and other conduct problems. Overall, the treatment effects were small; however, there was a large amount of variance due to differences across the studies examined.

- Programs targeted to at-risk populations showed greater improvements, meaning that prevention strategies were particularly effective with adolescents who were at higher risk for these types of behavioural problems.

- Treatment success also varied with the type of program used. Cognitive-behavioural or behavioural approaches that targeted self-control or social competency consistently showed positive results for all types of conduct problems, including substance use. This was true when these approaches were used individually or in larger groups such as entire classrooms. However, non-cognitive-behavioural counselling, social work and other non-cognitive-behavioural therapeutic interventions consistently showed negative treatment effects across all types of behavioural problems. This demonstrated that these approaches actually led to increases in problem behaviours. Mentoring, tutoring, recreation programs or community service programs were also ineffective at reducing problem behaviours.

- Two programs were particularly effective in the school system at reducing behaviour problems: Lochman's Anger Coping program and Bry's behaviourally-based prevention program. These programs target high-risk youths with services that use cognitive retraining and behavioural methods such as tracking of specific behaviours, behavioural goals and the use of positive and negative reinforcement to change behaviour.

SOURCE

Wilson, D.B., Gottfredson, D.C. & Najaka, S.S. (2001). School-based prevention of problem behaviors: A meta-analysis. *Journal of Quantitative Criminology, 17(3)*, 247–272.

Treatment

Which Treatments Do Harm?

This paper reviews two studies to clarify the findings of other studies suggesting that antisocial youth who are treated in groups with other antisocial youth are actually at risk for increased delinquent behaviour, substance use and violence.

Adolescent transition program study (ATP)

Youth at high risk were randomly assigned to four groups: parent focus, teen focus, parent and teen focus and a placebo group.

RESULTS

• The short-term results of all three treatment groups were positive, compared to the placebo group.

• The long-term results for the teen focus group were negative; there was an increase in substance use and delinquent behaviour.

• Three years later, these results persisted. Additional analysis showed that older youth who initially had a high level of antisocial behaviour responded more negatively to treatment.

The Cambridge-Sommerville youth study

In this study, high-risk boys were randomly assigned to a treatment or control group. Treatment started when boys were, on average, 10.5 years old, and terminated when they were 16 years old.

RESULTS

• The results, reported shortly after the program ended, showed that boys in the treatment group did no better than boys in the control group.

• Long-term follow-up results were more disappointing; the boys in the treatment group did worse than boys in the control group. A dose-response analysis showed that the boys who were in the program longer and received more intense treatment were actually more likely to have negative outcomes than other adolescents in the program.

COMMENT

Evidence indicates that when antisocial youth are treated in institutional settings their behaviour is more likely to be influenced by peers than by the staff. Therefore, the authors suggest avoiding treating antisocial youth in groups.

SOURCE

Dishion, T.J., McCord, J. & Poulin, F. (1999). When interventions harm—Peer groups and problem behavior. *American Psychologist, 54,* 755–764.

Treatment Effects on Children and Their Families

Most treatment studies for conduct behaviour problems have only looked at the effects on the child's functioning. The goal of this study was to also examine effects of therapy on child, parent and family functioning. Two hundred and fifty children, between the ages of two and 14, and their families were treated. Families with younger children received parent management training (PMT) alone. Families with children aged seven and older received either cognitive problem-solving skills training (PSST), PMT or a combination of both.

RESULTS

- In children, the symptoms that improved included disruptive behaviour observed in and out of the home, antisocial behaviour and symptoms in general. In parents, improved symptoms included less depression, stress and symptoms in general.

- Family relations and social support also improved over the course of therapy.

- Child improvements were greater than parent or family improvements.

- Those families who did not do well with treatment had lower incomes and had difficulties participating in treatment.

COMMENT

This is one of few studies that measure changes in parents and families as a result of the treatment of children for behaviour problems. This measure is particularly important because it would be difficult for a child to keep improving if the family were not functioning better. Interestingly, marital functioning did not change significantly with treatment. Finally, we still need to find ways to help the most disadvantaged and vulnerable families in society, as they tend to improve the least with therapy.

Source

Kazdin, A.E., Wassell, G. (2000). Changes in child, parent, and family functioning as a result of therapy. *Journal of the Academy of Child and Adolescent Psychiatry, 39(4)*, 414–420.

Treatment for Adolescent Sexual Offenders

Treatment programs for adolescent sexual offenders have increased significantly in North America over the past 20 years. However, despite the notable consensus regarding treatment goals, and the recent proliferation of treatment programs, little is known about the success of specialized treatment.

The objectives of this study were to determine:

- the success of specialized community-based treatment programs for reducing adolescent sexual offending

- the risk factors for sexual and non-sexual offending in adolescent sexual offenders.

Data such as criminal records were collected for 58 offenders participating in at least 12 months of specialized treatment at the SAFE-T program. Data were also collected from a comparison group of 90 adolescents. The follow-up interval ranged from two to 10 years, and offenders completed numerous psychological tests to provide data regarding social, sexual and family functioning.

Results

- Sexual re-offence was predicted by sexual interest in children.

- Non-sexual re-offence (violent and non-violent) was related to factors commonly predictive of general delinquency, such as a history of previous offences, low self-esteem, antisocial personality and economic disadvantage.

- No predictive variables were unique to violent non-sexual re-offenders; however, non-violent re-offences were additionally related to a negative family environment and perceived rejection by parents.

- Community-based treatment programs help to reduce the risk of adolescent sexual re-offence.

COMMENT

Some authors have questioned whether people who have committed a sexual offence are different from those who commit a non-sexual offence, and whether specialized treatment is effective for sexual offenders. This study supports the efficacy of treatment for adolescent sexual offenders and the notion that sexual aggression is related to factors that are unrelated to non-sexual offending. Comprehensive treatment that combines a strong family-relationship component with offence-specific interventions may be most successful for clinicians working with adolescent sexual offenders.

In this article the only predictive factor of sexual offence mentioned is sexual interest in children. Another related article states that a vast majority of sexual offenders have a history of being sexually abused and that the type of offending is related to how these offenders were themselves sexually abused. Therefore, past sexual abuse should be considered a predictive factor for sexual offending.

SOURCE

Worling J.R., and Curwin, T. (2000). Adolescent sexual offender recidivism: Success of specialized treatment and implications for risk prediction. *Child Abuse and Neglect, 24,* 965–982.

A Treatment Program for Delinquent Behaviour

Juvenile crime remains a national concern both in the United States and Canada. An estimated 2.9 million juveniles were arrested in 1997 in the United States, accounting for 19 per cent of all arrests. The high rate of incarceration of juvenile offenders is not only disturbing, but is also very expensive. It costs nearly $40,000 US to incarcerate a juvenile offender for one year, and conduct disorder is thought to be the most costly mental disorder. There have been many reports of cost-effective interventions, which reduce the rate of recidivism.

This study presents a one-year outcome of a short-term after-school diversion program for youth with delinquent behaviours. The study included 30 youth who completed the program:

- 55.3 per cent were first-time offenders, and the remainder were repeat offenders who had committed an average of 1.57 offences.

- The majority of the youths (84.1 per cent) had committed violent crimes such as assault and battery.

- Many of the youth came from low-income families, and 56.7 per cent lived in single-parent homes.

- 93 per cent were diagnosed with a mental disorder, 63.3 per cent had a diagnosis of conduct disorder, 23.3 per cent had attention-deficit hyperactivity disorder, 20 per cent had an anxiety disorder and 16.7 per cent had a depressive episode disorder.

The program consisted of youth meetings for two hours per day after school, four days a week for four weeks. Parents and guardians were required to attend 15 hours of the program. Consistent attendance was required both by the youths and by their parents, and if they missed more than three hours of the program, they were asked to leave. The program used a multitude of simultaneous treatment interventions. The project was called Back-on-Track (BOT).

RESULTS

- The youths who had completed the program committed significantly fewer offences than the control group at a 12-month follow-up (three offences compared to 21).

- The cost of the treatment per youth was $600, which was roughly the same as the cost of implementing and enforcing community control for the control group. Because the control group committed many more offences and the cost of each arrest and arraignment is approximately $3,000, the program provided considerable savings. There are of course the intangible savings of pain, suffering, fear and death.

COMMENT

The authors point out that the estimated monetary value of saving a high-risk youth from dropping out of high school and entering into a long-term criminal career is between $1.7 to $2.3 million. In spite of such findings, youths who display difficult and antisocial behaviour, grade after grade in school continue to get suspended instead of getting help for themselves and their families. We can reduce the number of jailed youth by identifying and helping high-risk youth in schools. We can also save a great deal of money and suffering in the long run.

SOURCE

Myers, W.C., Burton, P.R.S., Sanders, P.D., Donat, K.M., Cheney, J., Fitzpatrick, T.M. & Monaco, L. (2000). Project back-on-track at 1 year: A delinquency treatment program for early-career juvenile offenders. *Journal of the American Academy of Child and Adolescent Psychiatry*, 3(9), 1127–1134.

Home-Based Treatment for Youth in Psychiatric Crisis

It has been recognized that emotional and behavioural problems in children and adolescents should be treated in the home and should include the family and others who are involved with the youth. Multi-systemic therapy (MST) is a treatment approach that assumes that improvements in youth functioning are best achieved by favourable changes in the family, peer and school contexts.

Past research has shown that MST is an effective approach for antisocial youth and violent juvenile offenders. This study was designed to determine whether MST can be used as an alternative to inpatient psychiatric hospitalization for youths presenting with psychiatric emergencies.

There were 113 adolescents who were referred for psychiatric treatment. They were randomly assigned to either MST or psychiatric hospitalization. Most had disruptive behaviour disorders, including oppositional defiant disorder, conduct disorder and attention-deficit hyperactivity disorder. Some had a mood disorder, anxiety disorder, substance related disorder or psychosis. The average duration of psychiatric hospitalization was 3.8 days while youths in MST received care for an average of four months.

RESULTS

- MST was at least as effective as hospitalization for youth with internalizing symptoms (e.g., anxiety and depression) and more effective for youth with externalizing symptoms (e.g., aggression and noncompliance.)

- The complexity and severity of problems presented by youths and their families in psychiatric crisis were significantly greater than expected. Therefore, a substantial percentage of youths in MST were hospitalized for a brief period.

- Families of youths in MST showed improved cohesion and structure after the treatment, whereas the families of youths who were hospitalized did not. Also, youths in MST had greater school attendance than those who were hospitalized.

SOURCE

Henggeler, S.W., Rowland, M.D., Randall, J., Ward, D.M., Pickrel, S.G., Cunningham, P.B., Miller, S.L., Edwards, J., Zealberg, J.J., Hand, L.D. & Santos, A.B. (1999). Home-based multi-systemic therapy as an alternative to the hospitalization of youths in psychiatric crisis: Clinical outcomes. *Journal of the American Academy of Child and Adolescent Psychiatry, 38,* 1331–1339.

Wilderness Programs for Delinquent Behaviour: An Evaluation

Wilderness challenge programs for youth involve rigorous physical activities with others in an outdoor setting. Backpacking, hiking and rock climbing are some examples. The idea behind this is to promote the adolescent's self-confidence and self-esteem. This is accomplished by the youth mastering new skills, solving problems and working with others in a group.

This article examined 28 studies to determine if there was any impact on the rate of re-arrest for these youths. The authors also looked for aspects of the programs that were associated with better outcome.

RESULTS

- All studies showed positive results on recidivism.

- There was some reduction in the re-arrest rate (29 per cent) of wilderness program participants versus non-participants (37 per cent).

- There were positive effects on self-esteem and interpersonal skills.

- High-intensity programs employing strenuous individual and group activities tended to greatly reduce delinquency.

- Shorter programs (less than six weeks) tended to have better outcomes. The reasons for this finding need to be explained in future research.

SOURCE

Wilson, S.J. & Lipsey, M.W. (2000). An overview of the research on impact of wilderness challenge programs on the behaviour of delinquent youth. *Evaluation and Program Planning, 23*, 1–12.

School-Based Cognitive Behavioural Programs for Aggression

There were 226 children involved in this cognitive behavioural program, 183 boys (most of whom were under age 12) and 43 girls. The program ran for two months with 45-minute sessions every second day.

To move to the next stage, each child had to be successful at each of three stages:

- Acquisition: The children were taught specific skills that were modelled by the teacher, role-played by the students and reinforced by the teacher with tokens and praise when the children displayed appropriate behaviours.

- Transference: The teacher recorded whether children displayed the behaviours in the school setting during a specific time period. The teacher then gave the children tokens to reinforce these behaviours. Teachers were also instructed to give verbal praise and provide children with more social reinforcement than material reinforcement down the road.

- Generalization: The goal here was to help children use skills outside the reinforcement structure. They were only reinforced some of the time; they had to display the skills for the entire day to receive the reinforcement. To compensate for the increased difficulty of the task, the number of tokens used for reinforcement was increased.

Parenting

The parents of the children participated in a group modelled after the Systematic Training for Effective Parenting (STEP). These groups were held once a week in the evening. An important component in this treatment is the reciprocal relationship between the children and their environment. Parents must be involved in the treatment so they can continue reinforcing the child's good behaviours after treatment is completed.

RESULTS

- Aggressive behaviour was reduced in all cases.

- Reduced aggressive behaviour was more noticeable in boys who were unpopular and aggressive than in boys who were popular and aggressive.

- Although boys who were popular and unpopular had similar aggression scores after treatment, the unpopular boys may have shown more improvement because they were rated as more aggressive prior to treatment.

COMMENT

The authors suggest that children who are unpopular and aggressive have reactive aggression. This aggression is an angry response to perceived hostility. Thus, it is possible that unpopular boys showed greater improvement because they had more motivation to improve their social situation.

The article also suggests that children who are popular and aggressive have proactive aggression. Unlike reactive aggression, proactive aggression is used to gain social advantage. In this case, it would be hard to influence the popular aggressive children, as we would be asking them to give up the sources of their social influence and power. In addition, society also rewards and values proactive aggression—immense amounts of privilege can be obtained through its use.

SOURCE

Phillips, D.R., Schwean, V.L. & Saklofske, D.H. (1997). Treatment effect of a school-based cognitive-behavioural program for aggressive children. *Canadian Journal of School Psychology, 13*, 60–67.

Services for Families in School Settings

Evidence indicates that families influence the development of antisocial behaviour in adolescents. This study describes the Adolescent Transition Program (ATP), a multi-level family-centred intervention model delivered in middle-school.

The ATP model includes the following three levels: universal, which reaches all parents in the school setting; selected, which addresses the needs of at-risk families; and indicated, which provides family therapy as treatment.

Universal

The universal model recommends that the school have a family resource room, which helps school staff collaborate with parents. The goal is to offer information related to protective parenting practices, family management practices and to provide videotapes related to parenting during the teenage years. During the summer months, parents are offered home visits that focus on a "plan for success" for each student in the coming year. During the fall term, a consultant delivers six weeks of parent-child weekly exercises aimed at success at school and reducing substance use and conflict.

Selected

A three-session intervention offers family assessments and professional support and motivation to change. The three-session intervention includes the initial interview, a comprehensive assessment and a feedback session. Feedback must be presented in a supportive and motivational manner.

Indicated

The indicated model provides direct support to parents through various ways, including a brief family intervention, school monitoring system, parent groups, behavioural family therapy and case management services.

RESULTS

- Applying the indicated model reduced parent-child conflict, antisocial behaviour (as reported by teachers) and substance use.

- Follow-up studies have shown that the behaviour of children whose parents received family assessment improved compared to the families who did not participate.

COMMENT

Remarkably, the authors previously found that peer interventions led to an escalation in delinquent behaviour and smoking in school, though parenting interventions led to positive results.

SOURCE

Dishion, T.J. & Kavanagh, K. (2000). A multi-level approach to family-centered prevention in schools: Process and outcome. *Addictive Behaviors, 25(6),* 899–911.

Early Teacher-Child Relationships

Studies have shown that children who are able to successfully navigate early social environments in school get off to a better start and continue to profit from their social knowledge and experience as they progress through elementary and middle school. This study followed a sample of 179 children from kindergarten through Grade 8 to examine the extent to which kindergarten teachers' relationships with their students, as perceived by the teacher, are associated with children's academic and behavioural outcomes.

RESULTS

- Early experiences of teacher-child relationships marked by conflict and dependency are predictors of academic and behavioural outcomes through Grade 8.

- These negative experiences in teacher-child relationships continued to predict behavioural outcomes into upper-elementary and middle school.

- Negative experiences were also particularly evident for children with high levels of behaviour problems in kindergarten and for boys in general.

COMMENT

The authors suggest that these results have implications for theories of the determinants of school success, the role of adult-child relationships in development and a range of early intervention and prevention efforts. This study illustrates that a child's ability to form relationships with his or her teachers can predict later academic and behavioural adjustment in school.

SOURCE

Hamre, B.K. & Pianta, R.C. (2001). Early teacher-child relationships and the trajectory of children's school outcomes through eighth grade. *Child Development, 72(2),* 625–638.

Chapter 2
Aggressive Behaviour

Aggression

Direct physical harm, verbal harm, threat of harm or indirect harm (e.g., social manipulation, rumours, exclusion, ostracization and rejection) for personal gain or as a reaction to the hostility of others (actual or perceived). The scope of this chapter excludes self-directed aggression.

Characteristics and Related Issues

Youth Violence and Mental Illness

Are people with mental disorders at risk for committing violence? This study looked at a sample of young adults to find if there is an association between mental disorders and violence. The purpose was to inform strategies for preventing or limiting violence among people with mental illnesses.

The study included 961 young adults born in the same year who were measured for prevalence of mental disorders using standardized DSM-III-R interviews, self-reports of past-year violence and official conviction records. The following three hypotheses were also tested to explain the association between disorders and violence:

- Use of substances before offending: It is suggested that alcohol facilitates violence by disinhibiting aggressive impulses.

- Schizophrenia-spectrum disorder and perceived threat: It is suggested that psychotic delusions give patients strong subjective impressions of external threats that suppress self-control and may lead them to attack others.

- History of conduct disorder: It is suggested that children with conduct disorder who learn to use aggression at home generally use aggressive behaviour toward others as their social environments expand.

RESULTS

- People who had a substance dependence and/or schizophrenia-spectrum disorder made up 55 per cent of violent individuals in the sample.

- 11 per cent of the sample risk committing a violent offence because of alcohol dependence.

- 28 per cent of the sample risk committing a violent offence because of marijuana dependence.

- 9.6 per cent of the sample risk committing a violent offence because of schizophrenia-spectrum disorder.

- Having two or more of these disorders at once more than doubled the risk of violence.

- Among people with alcohol dependency problems, violence was best explained by substance use before the offence.

- Among people who were dependent on marijuana, violence was best explained by a juvenile history of conduct disorder (marijuana use alone does not precipitate violence).

- Among people who had schizophrenia-spectrum disorder, violence was best explained by excessive perception of threats and a history of conduct disorder.

COMMENT

People with mental disorders account for a considerable amount of violence in the community; however, not all people with mental disorders engage in violence. This study suggests that the link to violence is limited to the three diagnoses: alcohol dependence, marijuana dependence and schizophrenia-spectrum disorder. The authors suggest that the link between mental disorders and violence is often due to childhood and adolescent conduct problems, and therefore, primary prevention can be a solution.

SOURCE

Arseneault, L., Moffitt, T.E., Caspi, A., Taylor, P.J. & Silva, P.A. (2000). Mental disorders and violence in a total birth cohort. *Archives of General Psychiatry*, 57(10), 979–986.

Psychiatric Disorders in Aggressive Youth

It is very easy to diagnose oppositional defiant disorder or conduct disorder in a child. These terms simply illustrate whether a clinician feels the child meets criteria under the DSM-IV.

However, this study addresses, in a very practical way, how a clinician looks for the underlying causes of the child's antisocial and aggressive behaviour. The following diagnoses and conditions need to be kept in mind if one is to serve a child who is aggressive and violent. Any one or a combination of the following disorders when combined with physical abuse can be a recipe for violence. When an impaired child is abused, the child has a very high chance of becoming violent in adolescence or adulthood.

Attention-deficit hyperactivity disorder (ADHD)

Chief features of this disorder include impulsiveness, short attention span, cognitive and school difficulties, social skills problems, overactivity and poor judgment. Children with ADHD and early conduct problems are at a much higher risk for adolescent aggression and delinquency. Mood and dissociative disorders also have to be ruled out (see below).

Mood disorders

Mania in childhood or adolescence looks a lot like ADHD or conduct disorder. Episodes tend to be more variable, have mixed features (depressive and manic) and more "rapid cycling" (frequent mood switches) than in adults. Where there is clinical suspicion, especially when the person shows excessive energy, "workaholism" or gambling, it is crucial to look at family medical history, not just at the medical condition. Any agitated, aggressive or belligerent young person needs to have this condition ruled out or addressed.

Thought disorders

Extremely violent children can be psychotic or have more subtle paranoia, delusions or ways of thinking about the world. Auditory hallucinations are rarely volunteered and need to be inquired about in a delicate fashion. One way is to ask questions about physical health (vision, hearing, etc.).

Dissociative disorders

If children do not recall their actions, have features that resemble a seizure disorder (particularly complex partial seizures), appear moody, lie frequently, periodically hear voices, commands or arguments, they may have a dissociative disorder. Violent adolescents and children often have a tragic history of severe physical and/or sexual abuse or neglect. Dissociation is a way of coping with these overwhelming stressors.

Substance use problems

Alcohol and other substances (crack, PCP, amphetamines, heroin, benzodiazepines, barbiturates, anabolic steroids) are associated with violent crime or crimes related to drug use. Substances are often used to relieve the symptoms of ADHD, mood disorders, anxiety, psychotic disorders or dissociative states. They are also used to cope with the stress of living in difficult environments, families and conditions.

Learning problems

Violent youth tend to have a verbal IQ of eight to 17 points below non-violent youth. Various disabilities such as verbal, visual-spatial learning and reading are often associated with difficulties in reading social cues and thus poor social skills. School failure, truancy and underachievement are at least in part the result. Educational assessment is invaluable in these circumstances.

Executive functions

Executive functions include self-control in the areas of attention, concentration, abstract reasoning, anticipation, planning, goal setting and inhibition of undesired behaviour. Youth with multiple problems often have difficulties with executive functions. These difficulties frustrate adults, who end up reinforcing the antisocial styles of these youth; our current social expectations leave little room for understanding and assessing these difficulties.

RESULTS

- Success in treating aggression is achieved when attention is paid to the underlying psychopathology and not from just focusing on the aggression.

SOURCE

Yeager, C.A. & Lewis, D.O. (2000). Mental illness, neuropsychologic deficits, child abuse, and violence. *Child and Adolescent Psychiatric Clinics of North America, 9(4),* 793–813.

Aggressive Behaviour: Risk and Protective Factors

Risk factors

The following risk factors increase the likelihood of youth developing aggressive behaviour:

Individual

- male, non-white and older youths
- youth who lack adequate life skills, self-control and have low self-esteem

- youth with more favourable attitudes toward certain negative behaviours (e.g., fighting, drug and alcohol use)

Family environment

- use of violence to solve conflicts

- family disorganization, lack of family cohesion, poor parental supervision

- general absence of support, rules and positive expectations

School environment

- schools that are unsafe, dirty and that do not have consistent rules (as opposed to schools that are safe, well managed and have clear policies and rules regarding behaviour and general expectations)

- young people who experience academic failure at an early age and therefore are more likely to become distracted and withdrawn from the academic environment

General environment

- exposure to violence, either as witness or victim

Protective factors

Protective factors that reduce the negative impact of risk factors include:

Individual

- high IQ, resilient temperament, strong coping skills, high self-esteem

- bonding skills

- strong relationships with family members, teachers or other significant positive influences

Healthy beliefs and standards

- a set of clearly established rules and expectations

- understanding of both the benefits and consequences of behaviour

COMMENT

This report points out that one risk or one protective factor will not determine who develops aggressive behaviour. An interaction between risk and protective factors predicts the outcome. For example, a child who lives in a dysfunctional family can grow up to be non-aggressive if he or she attends a good school and the community has other positive resources.

This research emphasizes how important it is for youth to form a close, warm and confiding relationship with an adult who has positive attitudes. This relationship can protect the youth from many risk factors.

SOURCE

Fitzpatrick, K.M. (1997). Fighting among America's youth: A risk and protective factors approach. *Journal of Health and Social Behaviour, 38*, 131–148.

Characteristics of Aggressive Children in Residential Treatment

Aggressive behaviour in children and adolescents is currently the most common reason for referral to a residential treatment setting. In this study, 51 severely emotionally disturbed youth (28 male, 23 female) with a mean age of 13.3 years were assessed in a residential setting.

The following behaviours were present:

- verbal aggression: 97.1 per cent
- physical assault: 90.2 per cent
- property destruction: 60.8 per cent
- self-injuring behaviour: 49.0 per cent.

Patients who committed a high frequency of daily assaults were compared to patients who committed a low frequency of daily assaults. Factors that differentiated patients who committed a high average of daily physical assaults from those who committed a low average of daily assaults included:

- gender (boys committed a higher number of daily physical assaults)
- removal from the home environment because of aggression
- use of verbal threats, destruction of property and self-injurious behaviour
- experience of physical abuse.

Factors that did not differentiate children who committed a high average of daily physical assaults from those who committed a low average of daily assaults included:

- psychiatric diagnosis or neurological disorders
- IQ
- age
- ethnicity.

COMMENT

This study suggests that children who are likely to commit an assault can be identified upon admission to a residential treatment setting, so that special programs can be developed for them. However, as the authors point out, we still do not know the most effective ways for dealing with youth who assault—medication, physical restraint, time outs or a combination of these.

SOURCE

Connor, D.F., Melloni, R.H. & Harrison, R.J. (1998). Overt categorical aggression in referred children and adolescents. *Journal of the American Academy of Child and Adolescent Psychiatry, 37*, 66–73.

Causes and Contributing Factors

The Development of Persistent Criminal Offending

Research into childhood development has increased our understanding of various patterns of criminal activity throughout all stages of life. This has given rise to the emerging field of developmental criminology.

This study evaluated the impact of family environment, cognitive ability and early behaviour problems on the timing and frequency of juvenile delinquency and continued criminal offending. Researchers hoped to be able to fill gaps in our understanding of how to use developmental influences to make valid long-term predictions about criminal behaviour.

Researchers analysed a large sample of juvenile offenders who were committed to custody in 1964 and 1965 with a 20-year follow-up of arrest data.

They found clear patterns of association between chronic juvenile offending and persistent offending in adulthood.

RESULTS

- Adverse family environment, cognitive ability, early involvement with alcohol, early age of first arrest and the number of early arrests were all significant predictors of chronic criminal offending after ages 21, 25 and even after age 31.

- The timing of the first arrest is one of the most powerful predictors of chronic criminal activity.

- Juvenile offenders with more arrests were more likely to persist in adult criminal activity. For example, 91.2 per cent of the men with one juvenile arrest were arrested again after age 21 as compared with 67.2 per cent of the men with no arrest record before age 17.

Family environment

- Consistent with other longitudinal studies, it was found that young men who grew up in adverse family contexts were more likely to be arrested at younger ages and to have more arrests prior to age 17. Four factors were identified:

  - erratic, threatening and harsh or punitive parental disciplinary practices

  - low parental supervision

  - parental rejection

  - weak emotional bond between boys and their parents.

- The above factors at age eight predicted initiation of juvenile delinquency and adult crime.

Cognitive ability

- Low cognitive ability was significantly associated with frequencies of arrest after age 18, but did not predict offending during the juvenile years. Even after controlling for race, socio-economic status, test motivation and academic attainment, the link between low cognitive ability and adult criminal patterns holds. Self-reports of offending verify that the association is not simply due to a greater detection of less-intelligent offenders by police.

- Cognitive ability can be regarded as a component of resilience (a protective function), so that those with higher IQs may be more likely to explore legitimate alternatives to crime.

Early behavioural problems

- Adolescents who drink, smoke or use illicit drugs are significantly more likely to steal, get into fights and commit other delinquent acts. Problem substance use as well as early school termination may limit future job prospects and involvement in socially sanctioned activities.

- Antisocial tendencies developed in the home create difficulties at school and with peers. The person becomes isolated from positive relationships and institutions, thereby increasing the chance of criminal activity.

COMMENT

Many studies have verified that adverse family environments can harm a child's development and abilities. Harsh physical punishment and parental rejection are consistently associated with delinquency. Interestingly, harsh punishment and parental rejection are also implicated in lowered IQ (as much as 25 points), which is correlated with delinquency, as seen above. Children of authoritarian parents are not only rejected by their peers, they are rated more negatively by peers and teachers. This increases their chance of dropping out of school.

This study clearly shows that early juvenile arrest is a strong indicator of future adult criminal activity. This is one more reason to intervene early to effectively deal with antisocial behaviour in children and adolescents. Intervention could prevent juvenile arrests and may reduce adult criminal behaviour.

SOURCE

Ge, X.J., Donnellan, M.B. & Wenk, E. (2001). The development of persistent criminal offending in males. *Criminal Justice and Behavior, 28(6)*, 731–755.

Types of Aggression and Later Conduct Problems

While they may use different labels, many past studies distinguish between proactive and reactive aggression. Proactive aggression is goal-oriented. This type of aggression may be used to possess objects or to control others (e.g., bullying) and does not require provocation or anger. Reactive aggression, however, is often a response to provocation or perceived hostility. Research has established that these two types of aggression are distinct, although one person can posses both types.

This study examined whether proactive and reactive aggression differentially predict later problems, such as delinquency and disruptive behaviours (e.g., oppositional defiant disorders and conduct disorders).

The participants in the study were 742 boys who were part of an ongoing longitudinal study that started with 1,037 kindergarten boys from low socio-economic areas of a metropolitan city.

RESULTS

- The results of the study indicated that when boys were 12, proactive but not reactive aggression predicted delinquency and disruptive behaviours, such as oppositional and conduct problems. One explanation given for this finding was that boys with high levels of proactive aggression may associate with more deviant friends than do boys with high levels of reactive aggression, who are more isolated from peers.

- Further results indicated that when both types of aggression were present, high levels of reactive aggression weakened the link between proactive aggression and delinquency. However, high levels of reactive aggression did not moderate the link between proactive aggression and disruptive behaviours.

SOURCE

Vitaro, F., Gendreau, P.L., Tremblay, R.E. & Oligny, P. (1998). Reactive and proactive aggression differentially predict later conduct problems. *Journal of Child Psychology and Psychiatry, 39*, 377–385.

Maltreatment, Aggression and Peer Rejection

Over four years, 107 maltreated children were compared to a similar number of children without a history of abuse or neglect.

RESULTS

- Chronic maltreatment by parents was associated with increased aggressive behaviour, as well as with increased risk of rejection by peers. This rejection occurred over several years during elementary school.

- The rejection by peers was found to be due to the heightened level of aggression in the children. Therefore children who have endured harsh treatment in general, as opposed to being subject to any particular form of abuse, are at high risk for both aggression and peer rejection.

COMMENT

It is known that both maltreatment and peer rejection are risk factors for later violence in children. Thus, children who have a long history of parental abuse (four years in this study) deserve special attention, services and treatment to reduce their risk of concurrent and later behavioural and interpersonal problems.

SOURCE

Bolger, K.E. & Patterson, C.J. (2001). Developmental pathways from child maltreatment to peer rejection. *Child Development, 72(2)*, 549–568.

Prevention

Predicting Violent Behaviour in Youth

Although the rate of serious violent crime has been declining, high-profile school shootings highlight the need to identify youth who are at risk of becoming violent.

Past research has found three categories of risk factors for aggression and violence in children and adolescents: historical, clinical and contextual factors.

Historical factors

- school problems: including truancy and academic failure

- maltreatment or abuse: physical or sexual abuse and neglect

- family maladjustment: family conflict, parental criminality and poor bonding with family members

Clinical factors

- problem substance use

- risk taking and impulsivity

- negative attitudes: attributing aggression, lack of empathy and remorse

Contextual factors

- negative peer relations: gang involvement and delinquent peers

- poor parental management: extreme or inconsistent discipline

- neighbourhood crime

- lack of social support

- stress and loss

RESULTS

The paper states that the following principles should be used in conducting risk assessments of youth for violence:

- Conduct an assessment that is systematic and in accordance with some structured or guided scheme.

- Conduct a detailed inquiry into the history of violence.

- Consider base rates and the age of onset of violence. Base rate refers to the known prevalence of a specified type of violent behaviour within a given population, over a given period of time. Some rates may be very high and, therefore, the act may not be as serious when the base rate is taken into account. For example, in a national survey of high-school students in the United States, 46 per cent of boys reported being in a physical fight one or more times in the past 12 months. The age of onset is important, as violent behaviour is more likely to continue into adulthood if it starts before age 11 than if it starts in adolescence.

- Determine patterns and precipitants in past acts of violence, whether there is an increase or decrease in the severity or the frequency of violent acts and the factors associated with these changes.

- Situational factors are important and include people perceived by the youth as causing stress, such as family, peers or any specific type of individual or group.

- Receive a consultation if the situation allows it.

SOURCE

Borum, R. (2000). Assessing violence risk among youth. *Journal of Clinical Psychology, 56*(10), 1263–1288.

Predicting Aggression in Adolescence

RESULTS

- Kindergarten boys displaying high levels of opposition and hyperactivity are at high risk of physical aggression in adolescence.

- The only parental characteristics that predict aggression in adolescence are low educational attainment and teenage childbearing in the mother. These characteristics in the father had no predictive power.

SOURCE

Nagin, D.S. & Tremblay, R.E. (2001). Parental and early childhood predictors of persistent physical aggression in boys from kindergarten to high school. *Archives of General Psychiatry, 58*(4), 389–394.

Preventing Violent Behaviour in Youth

Juvenile violence has been an ongoing concern due to the magnitude and increasingly severe nature of the violence. Traditional treatment efforts have been directed at youth who have already become serious offenders. These approaches reach relatively few children and their families, are labour-intensive and have been modestly successful. Some risk and protective factors can be identified at an early age; therefore, prevention efforts can be implemented before serious violent behaviour develops.

Risk factors for violence include:

- low socio-economic status

- difficult temperament

- chronic illness

- more than one psychiatric disorder

- parental psychopathology.

Protective factors for violence include:

- good family structures

- prosocial peer groups

- supportive communities.

The following are examples of prevention efforts with varying scope:

- Universal preventive measures: These target entire populations and need political support. Such preventions include widespread programs to enhance prenatal care, maternal and infant care and nutrition and family management for preschool children and parents.

- Selective preventive measures: These target at-risk populations. The Houston Parent-Child Development Center program—for preschool children experiencing economic deprivation, academic failure, early behaviour problems and poor family management practices—led to fewer behavioural problems and better family management practices.

- Indicated preventive programs for young persons at imminent risk of behaving violently: These have been a focus of mental health professionals for many years. Individual interventions, including psychotherapy, have not been shown to be effective when used in isolation. In addition, single-event intrusive programs such as "boot camps" have not shown long-term success. However, broad family- and parent-based psychotherapeutic interventions in the grade school years have proven to reduce violence and related psychopathology.

IMPLICATIONS

- Exclusive individual child interventions for violent conduct disorders do not work. This suggests we need to change our focus from individual to community child and adolescent psychiatry.

- Psychiatrists who work with children and adolescents must seek opportunities to be leaders or team members in well-organized and well-funded community prevention efforts.

SOURCE

Rae-Grant, N., McConville, B., Fleck, S., Kennedy, J.S., Vaughan, W.T. & Steiner, H. (1999). Violent behavior in children and youth: Preventive intervention from a psychiatric perspective. *Journal of the American Academy of Child and Adolescent Psychiatry, 38,* 235–241.

Violence and Drug Prevention in Schools

This study describes prevention and intervention programs being introduced in two middle schools (grades six, seven and eight) in a southeastern American city that has high rates of violence, suspensions and expulsions. The programs were selected because of their proven effectiveness, and because they target factors (family, school, neighbourhood and peers) associated with antisocial behaviour in youth. The three programs being introduced to each school are described below.

Bullying prevention program

- establishing school-wide rules against bullying and other aggressive behaviours

- providing teacher in-services to raise the awareness of the issue

- developing classroom rules against bullying

- consistently enforcing rule infractions

- holding regular class meetings for teachers and students to discuss bullying and other aggressive behaviour

Drug prevention program (ALERT)

The program has two goals:

- to prevent non–drug users from experimenting with drugs

- to prevent experimental drug users from becoming regular drug users

To achieve these goals, classroom activities are organized to include role-playing, group discussions and viewing of videotapes to help youth develop resistance and problem-solving skills.

Multi-systemic therapy (MST)

Although the above two programs are proven to be effective, they are unlikely to reach those youth who are at the highest risk of using drugs and perpetrating violence, because such youth are seldom at school. Therefore, there is a need for a program aimed at intensive family and community-based treatment. MST focuses on the strengths of the family members and treats them as full collaborators in treatment.

RESULTS

- It is hoped that when the above three programs are combined, they will address all known risk factors for antisocial behaviour in youth.

SOURCE

Cunningham, P.B. & Henggeler, S.W. (2001). Implementation of an empirically based drug and violence prevention and intervention program in public school settings. *Journal of Clinical Child Psychology, 30(2),* 221–232.

School-Based Violence Prevention Program

School-based intervention programs have recently been implemented in many school settings in an effort to prevent youth violence. While there is little research on the effectiveness of these interventions, some intervention programs for young children have been proven effective. The objective of this study was to evaluate the effects of a prevention program delivered to almost 2,000 students in grades four through eight, called the Peacemakers program. A pre- and post-program assessment was done both on students involved in the program and on those who did not receive the intervention.

The Peacemakers program

This program includes a primary prevention component delivered by teachers. The intervention includes sessions related to attitudes about violence, values, and self-concepts.

The purpose of the primary prevention is to increase the attractiveness of non-violent behaviours and to strengthen the student's motivation to learn psychosocial skills (anger management, self-perception, problem-solving, conflict resolution, and peer pressure).

The second component of this program includes a remedial element implemented by school psychologists and counsellors for students referred because of aggressive behaviour.

RESULTS

- Evidence from student self-reports and from teacher-report measures indicated positive effects. The following six (out of seven) areas examined resulted in a positive change for students:

  - knowledge of psychosocial skills

  - self-reported aggressive behaviour

  - teacher-reported aggressive behaviour

  - number of aggression-related disciplinary incidents

  - use of conflict mediation services

  - suspensions for violent behaviour.

- The largest group difference, at 67 per cent, was reflected in a reduction in suspensions for violent behaviour. In other areas, intervention effects were stronger for boys than girls, and for middle-school students compared to upper-elementary-school students.

SOURCE

Shapiro, J.P., Burgoon, J.D., Welker, C.J. & Clough, J.B. (2002). Evaluation of the peacemakers program: School-based violence prevention for students in grades four through eight. *Psychology in the Schools, 39(1)*, 87–100.

Treatment

Treatments for Antisocial and Aggressive Behaviour in Children

RESULTS

Effective treatments

- Parent-management training: In this approach, parents are trained to change the behaviour of their children. Training is based on the perspective that many patterns of interactions between the child and the parent tend to promote the development of aggressive and antisocial behaviour. These patterns include rewarding non-compliant and aggressive behaviour by giving attention to it, inappropriately using negative consequences and harsh punishments and ignoring appropriate and approved behaviour. The objective of this approach is to alter the patterns of interactions between the child and the parent so that the parent is noticing and rewarding prosocial behaviour and ignoring or offering negative consequences for antisocial and non-compliant behaviour. This approach works best with younger children.

- Cognitive problem-solving skills training: "Cognition" refers to the way a person's mind perceives and experiences the world. It has been shown that aggressive children have deficiencies with various cognition patterns. For example, these children do not generate alternative solutions to interpersonal problems, they do not seem to know how to achieve goals such as making friends, and they do not foresee the consequences of their actions. In this approach, children are taught to engage in a step-by-step plan to solve interpersonal problems. Prosocial behaviours are taught through modelling and reinforcement. This approach is most suitable for children over the age of 10.

- Multi-systemic therapy: A child is influenced by many systems, such as family, school, peers and the neighbourhood. This treatment approach focuses mainly on the family, using many techniques, including parent-management training, problem-solving skills training and marital therapy.

Treatments that do not work

- Most of the treatments currently used in clinical practice, such as psychodynamic therapy, play therapy and relationship-based therapy, have not been well studied, and their benefits have yet to be demonstrated.

- There is also some evidence that treating youth with conduct disorder in a group setting could make them worse, because they seem to learn bad behaviours from one another.

- Therefore, it is better to use treatments that have been demonstrated to be effective.

SOURCE

Kazdin, A.E. (2000). Treatments for aggressive and antisocial children. *Child and Adolescent Psychiatric Clinics of North America, 9(4)*, 841–858.

Chapter 3

Conduct Disorder, Oppositional Defiant Disorder and Other Disruptive Behaviour Disorders

Conduct Disorder

A repetitive, persistent pattern of behaviour in which the person violates the basic rights of others or violates major age-appropriate societal norms or rules.

Oppositional Defiant Disorder

A pattern of negativistic, hostile and defiant behaviour lasting at least six months.

Disruptive Behaviour Disorder

Where youth do not meet the criteria of the two disorders above, but clinically significant impairment of behaviour occurs.

Characteristics and Related Issues

Conduct Disorder and Age of Onset

The DSM-IV (*Diagnostic and Statistical Manual of Mental Disorders*, American Psychiatric Association, 1994) classifies conduct disorder into two subtypes: childhood-onset and adolescent-onset. In childhood-onset type, at least one of the 13 antisocial behaviours characteristic of conduct disorder has to be present before age 10. In adolescent-onset type, the first antisocial behaviour occurs after age 10. The reason given for this subtyping is that early-onset cases are more likely than adolescent-onset cases to be male, aggressive and to have attention-deficit hyperactivity disorder (ADHD).

RESULTS

- This study suggests that in clinical practice it may not be easy to get a reliable age of onset of antisocial behaviour.

- When adolescents were tested and retested two to four weeks apart to determine the age of onset of antisocial behaviour, the responses were not the same. This was also true of information given by the parents.

- It was not possible to reliably predict the conduct of the children based on the subtyping.

COMMENT

The study's authors recommend that clinicians who use DSM-IV subtyping of conduct disorder be aware of its limitations. This subtyping depends on the adolescent being able to recall reliably and accurately the appearance of certain behaviours for the first time.

If clinicians use this subtyping, they should use multiple informants, focus on specific events and corroborate reports through school and other records.

SOURCE

Sanford, M., Boyle, M.H., Szatmari, P., Offord, D.R., Jamieson, E. & Spinner, M. (1999). Age-of-onset classification of conduct disorder: Reliability and validity in a prospective cohort study. *Journal of the American Academy of Child and Adolescent Psychiatry, 38*, 992–999.

Stability of Diagnosis in Preschool Years

Past studies have shown that problems in preschool years can remain stable for years. In this study, 510 preschool children were assessed three times over a period of four years. The age of the children at the first assessment ranged from two to five. The children were grouped into four diagnostic categories of disruptive disorders: oppositional defiant disorder, attention-deficit disorder, conduct disorder and a group of emotional disorders (e.g., anxiety disorder, depressive disorder). The diagnostic tools included questionnaires, an interview, a play observation and developmental testing.

Results

- A child with a *psychiatric disorder* diagnosed between the ages of two and five was two to three times more likely than a child not diagnosed with a disorder at that age to continue to have a disorder in the early school years.

- A child with a *disruptive disorder* was eight times more likely to have a disruptive disorder in the early school years.

- A child with an *emotional disorder* was four to six times more likely to continue to have an emotional disorder.

- From the data, the researchers predicted that a substantial number of young children (approximately 20 per cent to 30 per cent) who showed no signs of a disorder at preschool age would develop a diagnosable disorder over the next few years.

Comment

While it seems that some preschool children in primary care "grow out of" their disorder, an equally large number do not. This finding supports the need for early detection and intervention.

Source

Lavigne, J.V., Arend, R., Rosenbaum, D., Binns, H.J., Christoffel, K.K. & Gibbons, R.D. (1998). Psychiatric disorders with onset in the preschool years: I. Stability of diagnosis. *Journal of the American Academy of Child and Adolescent Psychiatry, 37*, 1246–1254.

Findings on Disruptive Behaviour Disorders

Many studies have followed children over a long period of time to determine adolescent and adult outcomes for children with disruptive behaviour disorders such as conduct disorder (CD), oppositional defiant disorder (ODD) and attention-deficit hyperactivity disorder (ADHD). This paper reviews findings over the last decade from a study started in 1987.

The study's aims were to:

- document the course of disruptive behaviour disorders (DBD) over time

- examine the interaction between DBD and other disorders (e.g., anxiety disorder) over time

- examine variables associated with the etiology (causes) of DBD.

Data were gathered on 177 boys referred to mental health clinics for DBD. The boys were aged seven to 12, with a mean age of nine and a half. They were followed up almost annually. Their parents and teachers were also interviewed on an almost-yearly basis. The following inclusion criteria were used: males aged seven to 12, not exhibiting a psychotic disorder, living with at least one biological parent and not an inpatient in a psychiatric hospital within the previous six months.

RESULTS

- Teachers were better informants than mothers and children on measures of inattentiveness and hyperactivity.

- Children with ODD were more likely to develop CD as they grew up.

- There appeared to be two developmental pathways to adolescent antisocial behaviour:

  - One group developed antisocial behaviour in late childhood or adolescence and indulged in infrequent, almost exclusively non-aggressive, antisocial behaviour.

  - The other group developed antisocial behaviour in early childhood and indulged in frequent aggressive and non-aggressive behaviours as they grew up.

Onset of symptoms

- As the child with conduct disorder grew up, the appearance of antiso-cial behaviours seemed to follow a sequence: The first symptom to appear in many children was cruelty to animals, followed by lying at home. More serious symptoms, such as firesetting, shoplifting and fighting, followed, appearing between ages six and nine.

Persistence of conduct disorder

- 88 per cent of children who met the criteria for conduct disorder in the first year of the study met the criteria again at least once in the three fol-lowing years. Thus, CD seems to show some persistence over time.

- The presence of antisocial personality disorder in a parent and low intelligence in the child increases the likelihood that conduct disorder will persist.

- Although this study did not show that the presence of ADHD affects the persistence of CD, other studies have demonstrated that ADHD is an important contributing factor in the persistence of conduct disorder.

Onset of ADHD and its symptoms

- The first symptoms of ADHD are hyperactive physical activity, which tends to appear between ages one and three, and inattention, which usually develops following hyperactive physical activity.

- The diagnosis of ADHD can be made between ages five and eight. The presence of aggression and behaviour problems suggests both short- and long-term persistence of ADHD.

- Hyperactivity and impulsivity tend to decline with age, while inatten-tion does not decline. Thus, certain ADHD symptoms seem to be more persistent than others.

Comorbidity (co-occurring disorders)

- 48.6 per cent of children who were diagnosed with ADHD in the first year of the study were also diagnosed with CD in later years.

- 61.8 per cent of boys with CD also showed symptoms of anxiety. The fact that most boys in the study were referred for psychiatric assess-ment may explain this high rate of comorbidity.

Substance use

The mean age for onset of

- alcohol use was 10

- smoking, around 13

- marijuana use, 15

- other drug use, also 15.

Physical fighting

- Nearly nine out of 10 fighters in the first year of the study continued to fight in successive years.

- One-third of the boys could be classified as long-term persistent fighters.

Academic achievement

- Boys with ADHD showed lower academic achievement than other boys in the study.

Family dysfunction

- 0 per cent of the boys with conduct disorder had a parent diagnosed with Antisocial Personality Disorder, compared to 23 per cent of the boys with ODD and 8 per cent of the boys in the control group (without CD or ODD).

- 28 per cent of parents of boys with conduct disorder were lax in supervising their boys with CD, compared to 20 per cent of parents of boys with oppositional defiant disorder and 8 per cent of parents of the boys in the control group.

- Disruptive behaviour disorders seem to have both genetic and environmental causes, though it is not possible to estimate the extent to which each factor is a contributor.

Maternal smoking

- Mothers who smoked more than a half a pack of cigarettes daily during pregnancy were significantly more likely to have a child with conduct disorder than mothers who did not smoke during pregnancy.

- The adverse effects, on the developing fetus, of maternal smoking during pregnancy may directly affect the development of conduct disorder. Alternatively, there may be other unidentified factors associated with maternal smoking that directly affect the development of CD. In any case, maternal smoking has a strong association with conduct disorder.

CONCLUSION

Children who are predisposed to disruptive behaviour disorders (e.g., those with difficult temperament and low intelligence) and also experience ineffective or abusive parenting or other adverse social interactions are at very high risk for developing conduct disorder.

SOURCE

Loeber, R., Green, S.M., Lahey, B.B., Frick, P.J. & McBurnett, K. (2000). Findings on disruptive behavior disorders from the first decade of the developmental trends study. *Clinical Child and Family Psychology Review, 3,* 37–59.

Abuse among Girls with Disruptive Behaviour Disorders

The objectives of this study were to determine

- the prevalence of physical and sexual abuse among clinically referred girls with disruptive behaviour disorders (DBD)

- differences in the prevalence of diagnoses and symptoms among girls with DBD who were abused and those who were not abused

- the age of onset of abuse and the onset of the first symptoms of conduct disorder.

Forty-nine clinically referred girls participated in the study. The mean age of the girls was 15.1. All of the girls were diagnosed with DBD, which included diagnosis of conduct disorder, oppositional defiant disorder and attention deficit hyperactivity disorder.

Families of the girls ranged across all five levels of socio-economic status (SES) as measured by the Hollingshead (1975) Four Factor Index of Social Status; however, 51 per cent of the girls came from the lowest two SES levels.

RESULTS

Prevalence

- 63.3 per cent had been physically or sexually abused.

- 30.6 per cent had been physically abused.

- 6.1 per cent had been sexually abused.

- 26.5 per cent had been both physically and sexually abused.

Diagnosis

- 86.7 per cent of the girls who had been abused had a diagnosis of conduct disorder, compared to 50 per cent of the girls who had not been abused.

- 53.8 per cent of the girls who had been both sexually and physically abused were diagnosed with major depression, compared to 11.1 per cent of the girls who had not been abused.

- 61.5 per cent of the girls who had been both sexually and physically abused had somatoform pain disorder (physical pain caused primarily from psychological distress, severe enough to impair daily functioning), while 6.7 per cent of the girls who experienced physical abuse only also had the disorder.

- Physical abuse appears to be associated with the development of DBD.

- Combined physical and sexual abuse are associated with internalizing disorders, such as depression and somatoform pain disorder.

Symptoms

- Truancy was the most common symptom for all girls examined.

- Truancy was present in 100 per cent of cases for girls who had been both sexually and physically abused.

- Truancy was present in 73.3 per cent of cases for girls who had been physically abused only.

- Truancy was present in 50 per cent of cases for girls who had not been abused.

- Girls who had been both physically and sexually abused had more internalizing symptoms (e.g., anxiety, depression) than did girls who had experienced physical abuse only or had not been abused.

Comorbidity

- Girls who had been both physically and sexually abused were more likely to have more than one disorder compared to girls who had experienced physical abuse only or had not been abused.

Age of onset

- 20 per cent of the girls in the sample had experienced physical abuse by the age of nine and 20 per cent had experienced physical abuse by the age of 10.

- The mean age of onset of any type of abuse was seven years.

- 40 per cent of the girls who had experienced both physical and sexual abuse exhibited their first symptoms of conduct disorder by age nine, as compared to only 10 per cent of the girls who had not been abused.

- Methodological difficulties in the study made it impossible to determine whether abuse preceded the development of conduct disorder or vice versa. This as an area for further research, given that earlier age of onset has been associated with later problem behaviour in studies of males.

Source

Green, S.M., Russo, M.F., Navratil, J.L. & Loeber, R. (1999). Sexual and physical abuse among adolescent girls with disruptive behavior problems. *Journal of Child and Family Studies, 8,* 151–168.

Predicting Conduct Disorder in Girls

Limited attention has been given to factors that lead to the development of conduct disorder in girls. This is true despite the fact that conduct disorder is one of the most common diagnoses for adolescent girls.

Results

- Girls with serious disruptive behaviour in kindergarten are prone to develop conduct disorder in adolescence; however, the incidence is lower among girls than boys.

- Only one in 12 girls in kindergarten with serious disruptive behaviour had a diagnosis of conduct disorder in adolescence, compared to one in eight boys.

SOURCE

Cote, S., Zoccolillo, M., Tremblay, R.E., Nagin, D. & Vitaro, F. (2001). Predicting girls' conduct disorder in adolescence from childhood trajectories of disruptive behaviors. *Journal of the American Academy of Child and Adolescent Psychiatry, 40(6),* 678–684.

Causes and Contributing Factors

Response Inhibition in Children with Disruptive Disorders

Executive functions include self-control in the areas of attention, concentration, abstract reasoning, anticipation, planning, goal setting and inhibition of undesired behaviour. These executive functions, mediated by the frontal lobes in the brain, allow people to inhibit or restrain themselves from inappropriate responses, and thus, contribute to adaptive functioning.

Research suggests that children with psychopathological disorders, particularly attention deficit hyperactivity disorder (ADHD), have trouble inhibiting responses. The objective of the present study was to determine whether response inhibition is unique to children with ADHD or is a component of other mental disorders.

Findings from eight earlier studies were combined to assess response inhibition in children with various mental disorders. All studies used a stop-task, a common measure to assess response inhibition. The child is given a task and then occasionally presented with a stop signal during the performance of the task. When the stop signal is presented, the child is required to break (inhibit) from the task. A measurement is taken of the time required for the child to inhibit a response after getting the stop signal.

In the eight studies, children were assessed in the following five groupings: children with

- ADHD

- Conduct disorder (CD)

- both ADHD and CD
- anxiety disorders
- none of these disorders—the control group.

RESULTS

- Impairments to response inhibition were present in children with ADHD, CD and both ADHD and CD.
- Children with both ADHD and CD did not show greater impairments than children with only ADHD.
- Children with anxiety disorder performed no differently from the control group.

COMMENT

The finding that children with ADHD or CD or both have impairment in response inhibition is not surprising, considering that the two disorders have many of the same symptoms. However, this finding does not necessarily mean that ADHD and CD reflect the same dysfunction. These disorders may share a general impairment in executive functions but have different underlying processes. At the present time, the mechanisms underlying impaired inhibition in child psychopathology are unknown. It is also unknown what conditions enhance or challenge the inhibitory control processes.

SOURCE

Oosterlaan, J., Logan, G.D. & Sergeant, J.A. (1998). Response inhibition in AD/HD, CD, comorbid AD/HD+CD, anxious, and control children: A meta-analysis of studies with the stop task. *Journal of Child Psychology and Psychiatry, 39*, 411–425.

Genetic and Environmental Factors in Conduct Disorder

There is still considerable debate over the role of genetic factors in childhood and adolescent conduct disorder. This study used a large population of male twin pairs born in the United States between 1940 and 1974 to investigate three questions:

- Has the prevalence of conduct disorder increased?

- Has there been a simultaneous increase in the number and types of symptoms in conduct disorder over the years?

- If the number and types of symptoms have changed in conduct disorder, have the underlying genetic and environmental influences also changed?

Identical and non-identical male twin pairs were recruited as part of a longitudinal study of the genetic and environmental risk factors for psychiatric disorder. The 2,769 twins in the study (mean age: 37) were interviewed. They completed self-report questionnaires about the presence of specific antisocial behaviours during adolescence and the amount of contact and similarity of environments during childhood between the twins (i.e., a measure of shared environment).

RESULTS

- The results show that the mean number and variation in conduct disorder symptoms increased systematically across birth subjects: more symptoms and more variability occurred among twins born more recently.

- Shared environmental influences, such as family structure and family income, rather than genetic or non-shared environmental influences, best explained the change in the nature of conduct disorder over time.

CONCLUSION

Changes in socio-economic and demographic factors that tend to be shared between family members may be responsible for the increasing rates of conduct disorder.

SOURCE

Jacobson, K.C., Prescott, C.A., Neale, M.C. & Kendler, K.S. (2000). Cohort differences in genetic and environmental influences on retrospective reports of conduct disorder among adult male twins. *Psychological Medicine, 30*, 775–787.

Mental Disorders in Low-Income and Homeless Youth

This study examined 94 children living in poverty, aged nine to 17. There were 41 children from homeless families and 53 children from low-income but housed families.

RESULTS

- 39 per cent of the homeless youth and 17 per cent of the housed youth had witnessed some form of violence either at home or in the community.

- Homeless youth had moved 3.7 times over a 12-month period compared to 0.7 times for the housed youth.

- 70 per cent of the homeless youth had changed schools in the previous year compared to 32 per cent of the housed youth.

- 17 per cent of the homeless youth had been physically abused and 22 per cent sexually abused, while 15 per cent of the housed youth had been physically abused and 6 per cent sexually abused.

- Homeless youth had almost double the rate of mental disorders in various categories than the housed youth.

- The most common mental disorder in both the homeless and housed children was disruptive behaviour disorder, which is characterized by lying, stealing, aggression and oppositional and defiant behaviours.

COMMENT

This study supports other studies that identify a strong link between low income and mental disorders. More specifically, it demonstrates the link between low income and antisocial and violent behaviour in children.

However, the fact that the homeless youth had double the rate of disorders compared to the low-income housed youth signifies that homelessness has its own risk beyond poverty. This finding is not surprising, considering that homeless youth have less stable home and school environments and see more violence as victims or witnesses than low-income youth who have homes.

SOURCE

Buckner, J.C. & Bassuk, E.L. (1997). Mental disorders and service utilization among youths from homeless and low-income household families. *Journal of the American Academy of Child and Adolescent Psychiatry, 36,* 890–900.

Hyperactivity and Reading Disability

Research suggests that children with hyperactivity often perform poorly academically, and children with reading disability often have hyperactivity. This study was designed to define the relationship between reading disability and hyperactivity. A large group of boys, ages seven and eight, were examined and then followed up nine years later.

RESULTS

- Reading disability, even when it persisted throughout the school years, did not lead to hyperactivity.

- Hyperactivity did not develop as a result of educational difficulties.

- Children with both hyperactivity and reading disability tended to be more defiant and antisocial than children with hyperactivity but no reading disability.

- Children with reading disability were more likely to have poor academic achievement in their school years than were children with hyperactivity.

COMMENT

The findings provided little support for the idea that persistent reading disabilities lead to the development of hyperactivity or that hyperactivity leads to the development of reading disabilities. The authors suggest that hyperactivity and literacy difficulties may have a common genetic factor or set of factors that act independently on these two aspects of functioning.

SOURCE

Chadwick, O., Taylor, E., Taylor, A., Heptinstall, E. & Danckaerts, M. (1999). Hyperactivity and reading disability: A longitudinal study of the nature of the association. *Journal of Child Psychology and Psychiatry, 40*, 1039–1050.

Parenting Practices and Conduct Disorder

Past studies have shown that the development of conduct problems in children is related to parental behaviours: in particular, a lack of adequate supervision and a lack of involvement in the child's activities. Other parental behaviours related to the development of conduct problems include inconsistent discipline, not providing enough positive feedback for appropriate behaviour and the use of physical punishment.

This study was designed to determine age-related variations in parenting practices and the effect on children's behaviour. The study involved 179 children and adolescents between the ages of six and 17. Participants were divided into three groups by age for data analysis: young (ages six to eight), middle (ages nine to 12), and adolescent (ages 13 to 17).

RESULTS

- As children became older, parents became less involved in children's activities and provided less positive feedback. These results were most significant as the children moved from the young to the middle group.

- Parental monitoring and supervision decreased markedly as the children moved from the middle to the adolescent group.

- The use of physical punishment declined as the children grew older. In the young group (six to eight), physical punishment was used 2.26 times over a three-day period. This rate decreased to 1.67 times for the middle group (nine to 12) and to 0.53 times in the adolescent group (13 to 17).

The following parental behaviours were associated with the development of conduct problems:

- lack of involvement with adolescents, which may reflect a general tendency to give more autonomy to adolescents but should be done in combination with maintaining involvement

- physical punishment (particularly in the middle group)

- lack of consistency in discipline (which was most marked in the adolescent group)

- lack of supervision and monitoring (more so for the middle and adolescent groups than the young group).

SOURCE

Frick, P.J., Christain, R.E. & Wootton, J.M. (1999). Age trends in the association between parenting practices and conduct problems. *Behaviour Modification, 23*, 106–128.

Prevention

Conduct Disorder: It Can Be Prevented

Studies have shown that early intervention programs to prevent antisocial behaviour in childhood and adolescence are most successful. Successful programs are intensive, have multiple components and target a largely disadvantaged population. Therefore, it would be most effective to reach children during their preschool years once they exhibit signs of antisocial and aggressive behaviour. This is meant to prevent aggressive behaviour during adolescence, which can be more difficult to treat. A number of prevention programs are available for children within the age groups under five, five to 11 and older than 11. The following programs have proven effective in the prevention of conduct disorder with the three different age groups:

Programs for children under age five

The Perry Preschool Project

This two-year intervention program was intended to promote academic, social and physical development in low-income, African-American children in the 1960s.

Trained teachers provided daily preschool and weekly home visits in an effort to help parents reinforce the preschool curriculum.

Long-term follow-up at ages 19 and 27 indicated important reductions in measures of antisocial behaviour for these children.

The Carolina Abecedarian Project

This intensive intervention program targeted the first year of life of an extremely high-risk group of children born to low-income, African-American mothers.

The program initially focused on using social services, medical care, home visits and parenting groups to improve language, perceptual-motor skills, social development and cognition.

From kindergarten to Grade 2, a home-school resource teacher helped parents with supplemental individualized educational activities for the child.

The results indicated that children who were involved in the full program did better on measures of IQ and school achievement than did children who were not, and children who received the intervention before age five had better results than those who began in kindergarten.

Prenatal and Early Childhood Nurse Home Visitation Program

The program results indicated that children whose mothers received home visits by a nurse during pregnancy and up to age two had more positive outcomes at age 15 than children whose mothers were not involved in the full program.

Youth involved in the full program had lower rates of arrest, convictions, running away, lifetime sexual partners and alcohol consumption.

Programs for children aged five to 11

Single-factor approaches

These approaches have been shown to have moderate effects in reducing antisocial symptoms. For an example, see the Good Behaviour Game. This game is based on the premise that antisocial youth have not been properly socialized. In other words, they have not been consistently rewarded for acceptable behaviour, nor had consistent consequences for unacceptable behaviour.

Multicomponent approaches

FAST Track program (as described on p. 115)

Competence-enhancement approaches

One example is the Seattle Social Development Project, aimed at developing social competence through teacher training in classroom management, child social skills development in Grade 1, child drug resistance in Grade 6 and parent training.

Results indicated that, by age 18, adolescents who had participated in the program reported fewer antisocial acts, less heavy drinking and fewer sex partners and pregnancies.

School development approach

This approach focuses on modifying and improving the school climate by using a planning and management team, a mental health team and a parent program.

Results showed superior school outcomes for those involved in the program.

Programs for children older than 11

Positive Action Through Holistic Education (PATHE)

In the PATHE program, a school team reviews and revises school policies, classroom goals are implemented through student participation and training, academic and climate innovations are effected school-wide, and academic and mental health services are made available for high-risk students.

Student reports indicate that this approach results in fewer antisocial acts and lower rates of drug use and school suspensions.

COMMENT

The review of various intervention programs for the different age ranges of children and youth illustrates that effective programs provide early intervention strategies and are intensive, comprehensive and individualized to the child's needs.

SOURCE

Bennett, K.J. & Offord, D.R. (2001). Conduct disorder: Can it be prevented? *Current Opinion in Psychiatry, 14(4)*, 333–337.

Early Intervention Reduces Behaviour Problems in Adolescence

Previous studies show that factors leading to adolescent conduct problems, depressive disorders and substance abuse disorders appear as early as Grade 1. Early learning problems are linked to later depressive disorders. Early aggressive behaviour is linked to later antisocial behaviour, criminality and heavy substance use. Risk for antisocial and substance abuse disorders increases when aggressive behaviour interacts with shy behaviour and attention or concentration problems.

This study sought to reduce the risk for problem substance use, depression and antisocial behaviour by targeting both early aggression and achievement. All Grade 1 children in a U.S. city were randomly assigned to either one of two preventive interventions or to a control group. The first intervention was classroom-centred (CC) and was designed to enhance the behaviour management skills of Grade 1 teachers. The second intervention was centred on a family-school partnership (FSP) program and was designed to improve parent-teacher interaction and parental skills in managing child behaviour. A non-intervention control group provided comparison data, and the results were assessed when the children were in Grade 6.

Classroom-centred intervention (CC)

Three strategies were used:

- curriculum enhancements in language arts and mathematics
- a weekly classroom meeting to enhance child social problem-solving in a group context
- the Good Behavior Game, a team-based behaviour modification effort that awards points for precisely defined good behaviour and deducts them for off-task, shy or aggressive behaviour.

Grade 1 teachers completed 60 hours of training before beginning the intervention and attended monthly support meetings thereafter.

Family-school partnership (FSP)

This intervention consisted of:

- training in communication and partnership building for school staff
- weekly home-school learning and communication activities
- nine 90-minute workshops for parents on child behaviour management, led by the Grade 1 teacher and school psychologist or social worker.

Sessions ran for seven consecutive weeks in the fall, with a booster session in the winter and another in the spring.

RESULTS

- At Grade 6 (or age 12), both CC and FSP children were significantly less likely to show conduct problems, meet the diagnostic criteria for conduct disorder or have had a suspension from school during the previous year.

- CC children showed significantly lower rates of mental health service need and use.

- FSP intervention parents appeared to reject their children less and be more involved in reinforcing activities than did parents who did not participate in either program.

- Overall, the CC intervention appeared to be the most effective of the two; however, the authors speculate that future studies may show that a combination of both interventions produces superior results.

COMMENT

This study shows that early success with authority acceptance, attention to task and social participation predicts good social adaptation at a later stage in development. In particular, social survival skills, which include the ability to monitor and manage one's own behaviour, may be critically important during the adolescent years. While the classroom-centred intervention needed a significant initial investment in the skills and resource base of Grade 1 teachers, this investment was rewarded by a reduction in problems and in their attendant costs well into the future.

SOURCE

Ialongo, N., Poduska, J., Werthamer, L. & Kellam, S. (2001). The distal impact of two first-grade preventive interventions on conduct problems and disorder in early adolescence. *Journal of Emotional and Behavioral Disorders, 9(3)*, 146–160.

Aggression Prevention and Intervention Programs

Studies have shown that young children who are victimized by their peers experience, among other things, peer relationship problems, emotional arousal problems and academic difficulties, during the elementary and middle-school years. There is also evidence that early aggressive behaviour can predict later antisocial behaviour (physical aggression, criminal behaviour and spousal abuse). Children who show serious forms of antisocial behaviour early on may be at risk for developing aggression in a pattern of progressive seriousness—beginning with milder forms of aggression, such as bullying, teasing and annoying others, and moving on to more serious forms of aggression, such as physical fighting, gang membership, assault, robbery and rape.

The following programs focus on prevention and early intervention strategies that lessen the milder forms of aggression in kindergarten, elementary and early middle-school-aged children.

Promoting Alternative Thinking Strategies program (PATHS)

The PATHS program is a classroom-based, universal prevention program (a program used with all children in the schools, not only the children considered high-risk or having behaviour disorders) that is implemented by teachers for elementary school-aged children. Its main objective is to help children in the mainstream and those with special needs (learning disabled, emotionally disturbed and mildly developmentally delayed) to develop appropriate problem-solving, self-control and emotional regulation skills. These skills are taught through discussions, directed instruction, modelling and videotapes. Parents are encouraged to teach these skills at home.

RESULTS

- Recent evaluation results of this program found a modest positive effect on measures of aggression and hyperactive-disruptive behaviours.

- Another one- and two-year longitudinal evaluation found the program had lasting effects on emotional understanding, interpersonal social problem-solving skills and teacher ratings of externalizing behaviours (i.e., aggressive behaviours, antisocial behaviours).

Second Step program

The Second Step program is also a universal prevention program used class-wide by teachers to promote social skills in children from preschool through middle school. The objective is to teach students skills such as empathy, impulse control and anger management. The main points of the program are emphasized through class discussions, role-plays, modelling, corrective feedback and positive reinforcement.

RESULTS

- Children involved in this program showed less physical aggression and more neutral, prosocial behaviours.

First Step to Success program

The First Step to Success program is a selective intervention program (a program that identifies and treats children who are high risk for aggressive behaviour). The program is an intensive classroom- and home-based early identification and intervention program designed to prevent kindergarten students who are disruptive and aggressive from developing anti-social behaviour patterns.

There are three components:

- a comprehensive screening procedure used to identify high-risk kindergarten students
- a classroom-based intervention designed to reduce the students' aggressive and disruptive behaviours and increase prosocial skills
- a home-based component used to strengthen parenting skills and improve home-school communication.

RESULTS

- Children involved in the program displayed a decrease in aggressive and maladaptive behaviours, as reported by the teacher.
- Teacher ratings of adaptive behaviour and classroom observations of on-task behaviour increased.
- The program worked equally well for high-risk boys and high-risk girls.

Anger Coping program

The Anger Coping program is a targeted intervention program (a program that treats children who are already having serious problems with aggressive behaviour) implemented by a mental health professional and a school counsellor. The program uses small-group work to help aggressive boys better understand and identify anger, increase problem-solving abilities and improve social interaction skills.

The program has been used primarily with boys eight to 14 years old, but has recently been adapted for use with boys five to seven. The program involves the use of a treatment manual and video and covers topics such as goal setting, perspective taking, social problem-solving, awareness of physiological arousal, self-instruction techniques and alternatives to conflict in situations.

RESULTS

- Results indicated that children involved in this program displayed a decrease in aggressive and disruptive behaviours and an increase in self-esteem.

- A three-year follow-up study indicated that participants in this program had lower substance use, more competent social problem-solving skills and higher self-confidence than the comparison group.

The Brain Power program

The Brain Power program is a targeted intervention program implemented by school staff members with extensive experience in small-group interventions for youth at risk. The objective is to reduce the tendency of aggressive boys to assume hostile intentions of classmates and show reactive aggression toward their classmates.

The program uses videotaped segments, role-playing and discussions to help students learn to make more accurate, less intentional, attributions in potential social conflict situations.

RESULTS

- Decrease in the tendency of aggressive boys to make hostile attributions toward others.

- Reduction in the overall level of aggression.

COMMENT

Teachers are generally the first professionals who are in a position to identify and intervene with behaviour problems in children. Schools are the best place, outside of the home, to teach social skills to young children to prevent the development of antisocial behaviour as they grow up. In present-day society, when both parents often work outside the home, schools must teach not only academics, but also necessary social skills to help prevent and reduce violence in schools and society.

SOURCE

Leff, S.S., Power, T.J., Manz, P.H., Costigan, T.E. & Nabors, L.A. (2001). School-based aggression prevention programs for young children: Current status and implications for violence prevention. *School Psychology Review, 30(3),* 344–362.

Parent-Teacher Training

The early onset of behavioural problems in preschool children appears to be one of the best predictors of antisocial behaviour for boys and girls in adolescence. Because conduct problems become more resistant to change over time, prevention efforts should start in the early preschool years.

Head Start is a mental health prevention and early intervention program. It targets socio-economically disadvantaged populations with high rates of risk factors for the development of conduct disorders. Previous research in Head Start centres showed that, when parents participated in the Incredible Years Parenting Training Program as a universal prevention program (a program used with all children in the schools, not only the children considered high-risk or having behaviour disorders), there were significant improvements in child behaviour problems and in parenting interactions with children. However, these improvements did not decrease the children's negative behaviours in the school setting.

This study attempted to provide and evaluate a more comprehensive intervention program with the Head Start centres. The researchers hypothesized that the improvements in school behaviours were not seen in the original Head Start study because teachers were not given skills training in classroom management. In this study, researchers implemented and evaluated two empirically validated programs for treating children with behavioural problems (Incredible Years: Parent Training Program and Teacher Training Program) in Head Start classrooms.

The study involved 272 Head Start mothers and their four-year-old children and 61 Head Start teachers in 34 classrooms. Participants were randomly assigned to either the treatment group that received parent and teacher prevention programming for 12 weeks or to the control group that received the regular Head Start program.

RESULTS

- Mothers in the treatment group had significantly lower negative parenting scores and higher positive parenting scores than mothers in the control group.

- Children in the treatment group showed fewer conduct problems at home and at school than children in the control group.

- In addition, the teachers in the treatment group had better classroom management skills than did teachers in the control group.

- At follow-up, one year later, clinically significant reductions in serious behaviour problems for the children in the treatment group were maintained at home and at school.

SOURCE

Webster-Stratton, C., Reid, M.J. & Hammond, M. (2001). Preventing conduct problems, promoting social competence: A parent and teacher training partnership in Head Start. *Journal of Clinical Child Psychology, 30(3),* 283–302.

Nurse Home-Visitation, Maltreatment and Early Onset Behaviour Problems

Considerable evidence suggests that people who start committing antisocial or criminal acts before age 15 tend to commit more offences over a longer period of time than those who commit their first offence at a later stage. Studies show that a history of problematic parenting practices can be related to early-onset (EO) behaviour problems in children.

This study looked at the relationship between child maltreatment and the early onset of behaviour problems (criminal activity, substance use and sexual activity). The study also determined whether a nurse home-visitation program for low-income and unmarried mothers having their first child would prevent the development of EO problem behaviours. If the children of nurse-visited mothers were maltreated, the study then determined whether these children were likely to develop an early pattern of behaviour problems.

Participants were placed in the Elmira Nurse Home-Visitation Program or in a comparison group. Home-visitation services continued over a two-year period, and results were drawn from a follow-up study that took place when the children were 15 years old.

RESULTS

- The results of the comparison group indicate that child maltreatment is associated with an increase in the number of EO problem behaviours.

- The nurse-visitation program had two beneficial effects: it reduced the number of maltreatment reports and prevented the prevalence of multiple types of maltreatment; where maltreatment did occur, it prevented the maltreatment from becoming chronic.

SOURCE

Eckenrode, J., Zielinski, D., Smith, E., Marcynyszyn, L.A., Henderson, C.R, Kitzman, H., Cole, R., Powers, J. & Olds, D.L. (2001). Child maltreatment and the early onset of problem behaviors: Can a program of nurse home visitation break the link? *Development and Psychopathology, 13(4)*, 873–890

Treatment

Parents' Perception of Treatment and Treatment Outcome

Past research shows that certain factors predict poor treatment outcome for youth with conduct disorder. These factors include:

- low socio-economic status
- single-parent family status
- parent dysfunction
- severity of child dysfunction.

This study investigated whether parents' perceptions and experiences during the child's treatment affected the treatment outcome of youth with conduct disorder. Four factors that the parents perceived as affecting the treatment outcome of their child were investigated. These factors were:

- stressors and obstacles (conflict with the other parent about coming to treatment, parents' problems with their other children)

- treatment demands and issues (treatment perceived as confusing, too long, costly, difficult or demanding)

- perceived relevance of treatment (parents' perception of treatment as relevant to the child's problem)

- relationship with the therapist.

RESULTS

- The two factors most strongly related to treatment outcome were perceived relevance of treatment and treatment demands.

- Stressors and obstacles and relationship with the therapist also affected treatment outcome.

COMMENT

This study gives reasons why parents of children with conduct disorder drop out of treatment or fail to get involved. Very often therapists ask questions that parents view as irrelevant (e.g., issues related to the parents' childhood). Parents must be given reasons for such questioning (i.e., explain to parents that their own childhood often affects the way they raise their children).

Therapists should understand and appreciate the difficulties and stress parents may experience when they are asked to alter their behaviour toward their child. Most parents come to therapy expecting that the therapist will change the child's behaviour without making demands on them. By closely monitoring the response of parents to therapy, therapists will reduce treatment dropout rates and achieve greater involvement of parents.

SOURCE

Kazdin, A.E. & Wassell, G. (1999). Barriers to treatment participation and therapeutic change among children referred for conduct disorder. *Journal of Clinical Child Psychology, 28,* 160–172.

Family Therapy for Conduct Disorders

Approximately five per cent of children in the general population and 50 per cent of youth referred for treatment for behaviour problems have conduct disorder. Family dysfunction is one of the main contributors to the development of conduct disorder. Therefore, family therapy is used and has proven successful in treating conduct disorder. Family therapy can be applied in different ways. The following approaches to family therapy have proven successful in treating conduct disorder:

Structural family therapy

Minuchin, the main contributor to this approach, suggested that families of children with antisocial behaviour problems fall into two types: enmeshed and disengaged. In enmeshed families, antisocial behaviour is the result of the parent's and child's inability to separate, though they resent this dependency. In disengaged families, antisocial behaviour results when parents lack involvement with the child and do not set limits. Minuchin describes the actual mode of treatment in detail in his book, *Structural Family Therapy.*[1]

Functional family therapy

This approach encourages family members to examine the "function" of the conduct problems within the family. It aims to enhance support, positive reinforcement and reciprocity among family members and to establish clear interpersonal communication and negotiation to solve problems. Evaluation shows that this approach lowers the rate of recidivism and, in addition, the siblings of the youth with conduct problems showed lower rates of referral to the juvenile courts.

Behavioural family therapy

In this approach, the focus is the aggressive behaviour of the adolescent. The development of aggressive behaviour is related to high levels of parental conflict, lack of differentiation between the role of parents and children and the predominance of hostile and oppressive emotion in the family. Treatment should be focused on supporting a functional parent-child hierarchy and parental authority.

---

1. Minuchin, S. (1981). *Structural Family Therapy.*
   New York: International Universities Press.

Psychodynamic family therapy

This approach suggests that the child's antisocial behaviour is related to the parent(s)'s wish to have the child act as an agent for their own unacceptable tendencies and actions. Therapy should focus on issues related to neglect and abandonment, sexual and physical abuse, parental failure to create a holding environment for the child in the early years and parental conflict. There is no research-based evidence indicating that it is effective.

Other

Other approaches use family work as a critical part of treatment, such as multi-systemic therapy and parent management training. Both of these approaches have been shown to be effective.

SOURCE

Sholevar, G.P. (2001). Family therapy for conduct disorders. *Child and Adolescent Psychiatric Clinics of North America, 10(3)*, 501–517.

Child Training Program Produces Good Results

Parent training programs are an important treatment approach for reducing aggressive and non-compliant behaviour in children, but a number of limitations exist:

- Some parents cannot or will not participate because of work conflicts, life stress, personal psychopathology or lack of motivation.

- Some parents find it hard to implement or maintain the strategies taught because of interpersonal and family issues.

- About one-third of children with conduct problems whose parents received training continued to have peer relationship problems and academic and social difficulties two to three years later.

These shortcomings led to the treatment approach under review: directly training children in social skills, problem solving and anger management to address the cognitive and behavioural deficits known to be present in young people with conduct problems.

Families of 99 referred children, aged four to eight and with early-onset conduct problems, were randomly assigned to either a child training treatment group (CT) using the Incredible Years Dinosaur Social Skills and Problem Solving curriculum or a waiting-list control group (CON). Before treatment, three risk factors were assessed: *family stress* (maternal depression, marital discord, negative life stress, low income), *negative parenting* (harsh discipline such as maternal critical statements and physical force) and *hyperactivity* (attention-deficit hyperactivity disorder).

RESULTS

- The CT children had significantly fewer externalizing problems (i.e., aggressive behaviours, antisocial behaviours) at home, less aggression at school, more prosocial behaviour with peers and more positive conflict-management strategies than CON children.

- The CT children showed improvements both on reports and on independent observations of aggressive and non-compliant behaviour.

- Children's progress was evaluated with the three risk factors (hyperactivity, parenting discipline practices, and family risk factors). The only risk factor related to the failure to find improvements in child conduct problems after treatment was negative parenting.

- Neither an ADHD classification nor hyperactivity prevented gains for identified children.

- Remarkably, 80 per cent of the children who met the ADHD classification at the outset no longer met this classification at follow-up. This finding supports the theory that the co-occurrence of ADHD and conduct problems signals a shared underlying mechanism—parental discipline practices.

- Children with conduct problems whose parents had positive skills seemed to benefit from the added child training, even if they also showed ADHD symptoms, whereas those who still had negative and punitive interactions modelled at home were less likely to succeed with the child training alone.

- One-year follow-up showed that gains were maintained for CT children, while symptoms for untreated CON children worsened.

COMMENTS

This study shows it is possible to help children with conduct problems without involving the parents in therapy. This is very positive, as many families are either unwilling or unable to join the child's therapy. However, considerable evidence in almost all cases shows improved results when the family is involved. Therefore, every effort should be made to involve the parents whenever possible.

SOURCE

Webster-Stratton, C., Reid, J. & Hammond, M. (2001). Social skills and problem-solving training for children with early-onset conduct problems: Who benefits? *Journal of Child Psychology and Psychiatry and Allied Disciplines*, 42(7), 943–952.

Effective Treatments for Conduct Disorder

The following four programs have been found to be effective with children and adolescents with conduct disorder:

Behavioural management programs

The theory behind these programs is simple: youth with antisocial behaviour problems have not been properly socialized; that is, they have not been exposed to an environment where acceptable behaviour was consistently rewarded and unacceptable behaviour was given consistent consequences. Therefore, they have not learned to obey and respect other people's rights. In applying these programs, the goals of treatment have to be clearly defined, and rewards and consequences for chosen behaviour must be consistent, to achieve the desired behaviour changes.

These programs appear simple, but they have to be individualized so that goals are reasonable and rewards and consequences are likely to motivate the child.

Parent management training

The goal of this approach is to train parents to carry out a behavioural program in the home by teaching them more effective discipline strategies. It also aims to improve the quality of child-parent relationships so parents become more involved in their children's activities, thereby improving child-parent communication.

Cognitive-behavioural skills training (CBST)

Children and adolescents with conduct disorder have deficits in the way they process information; they misinterpret social cues and develop inappropriate responses. For example, if a peer acts in a way that is ambiguous (i.e., neither clearly friendly nor clearly hostile) the child with conduct disorder will assume the intent is hostile and act aggressively toward the peer. Children and adolescents with conduct disorder also tend to believe in positive outcomes from aggressive behaviour and consequently choose aggression when non-aggressive behaviour would have solved the problem better.

Most CBST programs take a child through a series of steps to solve problems, such as how to recognize problems, how to consider alternative responses and how to select the most effective response to the problem. The therapist plays a very active role, modelling the skills being taught, role-playing social situations with the child, prompting for the skills and delivering feedback and praise for using appropriate skills.

Stimulant medication

Many children who have conduct disorder also have attention-deficit hyperactivity disorder (ADHD). These children need a stimulant medication in addition to any of the above programs. Impulsivity is one of the characteristics of ADHD that leads to aggressive behaviour. Stimulant medication has been shown to be the most effective way of controlling the symptoms of ADHD.

Limitations of the approaches

- These treatment approaches are effective, but not in all cases.

- The treatments outlined are more effective with younger children than with adolescents.

- These approaches may be effective in one setting but not in other settings.

- The improvements brought about may not last.

- There may not be one single best treatment for conduct disorder.

Given that antisocial and violent behaviours may develop from such varied factors, and the reasons may vary from child to child, the approaches that are most likely to succeed will be individualized and comprehensive. The following programs have these two characteristics:

FAST Track program

The program aims to change children's environments at home and school. It also identifies and improves any deficits the child may have in social skills or academic learning. The program can be individualized and it is comprehensive. It has been used for children in Grade 1 and has five components:

- parent training, which is done in groups and focuses on teaching parental skills

- home visiting, which takes place twice a week and supplements the parent training

- social skills training to improve the child's social skills and peer relations

- academic tutoring to improve the child's reading skills

- classroom intervention to train classroom teachers.

Multi-systemic therapy

This approach focuses on many systems that may affect the child, such as school, peers and the neighbourhood environment, but the primary focus is on the family. Working with the family, this approach uses a variety of techniques, such as joining, reframing and enactments. The main goal is to build cohesion and emotional warmth among family members.

Many other approaches may be incorporated, if indicated, such as problem solving, skills training, parent management training and marital therapy. This program meets the requirements for being individualized (the therapist can use as many or as few techniques as required) and comprehensive (it focuses on any or all of the environments of the child as needed).

SOURCE

Frick, P.J. (2001). Effective interventions for children and adolescents with conduct disorder. *Canadian Journal of Psychiatry, 46(7)*, 597–608.

Effective Psychosocial Treatments for Youth with Conduct Disorder

The purpose of this review was to evaluate the literature on psychosocial treatment outcomes for children and adolescents with conduct problems and to identify effective treatments. A conduct problem was defined as any behaviour listed in the DSM-IV as a symptom of oppositional defiant disorder (ODD), conduct disorder (CD) or similar problem behaviours, such as temper tantrums, disruptive classroom behaviour or antisocial behaviour. Eighty-two studies from 1966 to 1995 were identified and coded according to the following criteria:

- Treatments identified as "well established" had several studies supporting the findings, including studies that met stringent criteria for the quality of the research methods, and no studies were found that disagreed with the data.

- Treatments identified as "probably efficacious" were supported by at least two studies showing that the treatment was more effective than a wait-list control or they were supported by a study meeting all the criteria for a well-established treatment, except replication by an independent research team.

In this review, two interventions met the criteria for well-established treatments and 10 treatments met the criteria for probably efficacious treatments.

Well-established treatments

Parent training programs

These treatment programs are:

- based on Patterson and Gullion's (1968) manual *Living with Children*

- based on operant (reward and punishment) principles of behaviour change

- designed to teach parents to monitor targeted problem behaviours, monitor and reward incompatible behaviours and ignore or punish the problem behaviours

- generally short-term behavioural parent-training programs.

Videotape modelling parent training

This treatment approach, based on Webster-Stratton's parent training program, includes a videotape series of parent training lessons and is for use in parent groups with therapist-led group discussion of the videotape lessons.

Parents receiving videotape modelling training:

- rate their children as having fewer problems after treatment than do the parents of the children in the control group

- rate themselves as having improved attitudes toward their children and greater self-confidence in their parenting role

- show better parenting skills than parents in the control group on observational measures in the home.

The children of parents who receive this training show greater reduction in observed deviant behaviour.

Probably efficacious treatments

Preschool-aged children with conduct disorder

Parent-child interaction therapy:

- Eyberg, Boggs & Algina (1995)
- McNeil, Eyberg, Eisenstadt, Newcomb & Funderburk (1991)
- Zangwill (1983)

Parent training program:

- Wells & Egan (1988)
- Peed, Roberts & Forehand (1977)

Time-out plus signal seat treatment:

- Hamilton & MacQuiddy (1984)

School-aged children with conduct problems

Problem-solving skills training:

- Kazdin, Siegel & Bass (1992)
- Kazdin, Esveldt-Dawson, French & Unis (1987b)
- Kazdin, Esveldt-Dawson, French & Unis (1987a)

Anger coping therapy:

- Lochman, Burch, Curry & Lampron (1989)
- Lochman, Lampron, Gemmer & Harris (1984)

Adolescents with conduct disorder

Anger control training with stress inoculation:

- Feindler, Mariott & Iwata (1984)
- Schichter & Horan (1981)

Assertiveness training:

- Huey & Rank (1984)

Delinquency prevention program:

• Trembley, Pagani-Kurtz, Masse, Vitaro & Phil (1995)

• Vitaro & Tremblay (1994)

Multi-systemic therapy:

• Borduin, Mann, Cone, Henggeler, Fucci, Blaske & Williams (1995)

• Henggeler, Melton & Smith (1992)

• Henggeler, Rodick, Borduin, Hanson, Watson & Urey (1986)

Rational-emotive therapy:

• Block (1978)

COMMENT

This review is a careful evaluation of the studies that report results of treatment for youth with conduct disorder. It should serve as an excellent guide to selecting treatment. If a treatment is not cited in one of the two categories (well-established or probably efficacious), its use should be justified, particularly among clinicians who believe in evidence-based practice.

SOURCE

Brestan, E.V. & Eyberg, S.M. (1998). Effective Psychosocial Treatments of Conduct-Disordered Children and Adolescents: 29 Years, 82 Studies, and 5,272 Kids. *Journal of Clinical Child Psychology, 27*, 180–189.

Chapter 4
Attention-Deficit Hyperactivity Disorder (ADHD)

Attention-Deficit Hyperactivity Disorder (ADHD)

Previously referred to as attention-deficit disorder (ADD), this disorder has three main symptoms: inability to concentrate, hyperactivity and impulsivity.

Characteristics and Related Issues

ADHD: Causes and Contributing Factors

Neuroimaging

- Recent advances in technology allow us to study the structure and function of the human brain as it actually functions in a living person. This is giving us a new understanding of developmental neuropsychiatric disorders, including evidence that fronto-striatal networks in the brain may be involved in ADHD.

Genetic studies

- Twin and adoption studies support the notion that ADHD is a disorder that is passed on from one generation to the next.

- These studies suggest that ADHD is caused by a number of genes rather than a single gene.

Comorbidity

- An estimated 50 to 80 per cent of children with ADHD also have other disorders.

- The most common disorders associated with ADHD are oppositional defiant disorder and conduct disorder.

- 15 to 20 per cent of children with ADHD also have a mood disorder; 25 per cent have anxiety disorders; and 20 per cent have learning disabilities.

SOURCE

Tannock, R. (1998). Attention deficit hyperactivity disorder: Advances in cognitive, neurobiological, and genetic research. *Journal of Child Psychology and Psychiatry, 39,* 65–99.

ADHD and Oppositional Defiant Disorder

Attention-deficit hyperactivity disorder (ADHD) is characterized by behaviour that is impulsive, hyperactive and inattentive. Previous research has established three main types of ADHD: (1) primarily inattentive; (2) primarily impulsive and hyperactive; and (3) combined impulsivity, hyperactivity and inattentiveness. The first type exhibits more appropriate behaviour and less aggressive behaviour than the second and third types.

RESULTS

- In this study, children with combined ADHD and oppositional defiant disorder (ODD) were found to have more problems than children with only one of these disorders.

- Results indicated that children with combined ADHD/ODD have more:
  - externalizing problems (i.e., aggressive behaviours, antisocial behaviours)
  - internalizing problems (i.e., anxiety, depression, somatic complaints)
  - social problems
  - attention problems.

SOURCE

Carlson, C.L., Tamm, L. & Gaub, M. (1997). Gender differences in children with ADHD, ODD, and co-occurring ADHD/ODD identified in school populations. *Journal of the American Academy of Child and Adolescent Psychiatry, 36*, 1706–1714.

ADHD and Mood Disorders

Researchers are becoming increasingly aware of the comorbidity (or co-occurrence) of disorders. This is particularly important as the comorbidity of disorders with attention-deficit hyperactivity disorder (ADHD) dramatically affects prognosis, treatment and health care delivery decisions. However, these comorbid disorders often share many of the same symptoms, which raises the question: Are comorbid disorders different expressions of the same disorder or are they separate clinical entities?

This paper examines the overlap of mood disorders, such as depression and mania, with ADHD.

Depression and ADHD

Children with ADHD often feel demoralized when in remission from ADHD, which makes it unclear if depression in children with ADHD is "true" depression or demoralization associated with ADHD. However, a longitudinal study of children with both ADHD and depression found that ADHD and depression had independent and distinct courses.

RESULTS

- Depression associated with ADHD is a depressive disorder, not merely demoralization.

- Research also suggests that children with both ADHD and mood disorders are at a higher risk of developing a wide range of impairments that affect multiple domains of psychopathology and interpersonal and family functioning.

- Relatives both of children with ADHD and of children with ADHD *and* depression had high rates of ADHD and depression compared with relatives of the children who had neither disorder.

- Researchers concluded that ADHD and depression may share common causal factors in relation to family genetics.

COMMENT

When prescribing medication to manage the symptoms of ADHD in children with comorbid depression/anxiety, it is particularly important to identify the comorbid disorders. For example, stimulants are normally used with children with ADHD to help reduce symptoms; however, when ADHD is accompanied by depression or anxiety, the ADHD symptoms may not respond as well to stimulants, and in some patients, stimulants may induce depression.

Bipolar disorder and ADHD

Bipolar disorder is a mood disorder characterized by mood swings from mania (abnormally elevated, expansive or irritable mood) to depression. In children with ADHD, mania is hard to diagnose because it is characterized by severe irritability, rather than euphoria (euphoria being more typical in adult mania). Mania and ADHD also share many of the same symptoms (e.g., distractibility, impulsivity, hyperactivity).

RESULTS

- Research suggests that children with ADHD are at greater risk of developing bipolar disorder, a severe disease causing great dysfunction and incapacitation.

COMMENT

The accurate diagnosis of these conditions may have major clinical consequences. For instance, symptoms of mania in children with ADHD can be controlled by mood stabilizers but not by stimulants or antidepressants (which reduce ADHD symptoms).

The authors state that, "Given the evidence of comorbidity of ADHD with major depression and bipolarity, ADHD children should be routinely examined for the presence of these comorbid conditions as these have clinical implications for diagnosis, prognosis, treatment and healthcare." In addition, "a careful family history may uncover a history of mood disorders among immediate relatives."

SOURCE

Spencer, T., Biederman, J., Wozniak, J. & Wilens, T. (2000). Attention deficit hyperactivity disorder and affective disorders in childhood: Continuum, comorbidity or confusion. *Current Opinion in Psychiatry, 13,* 73–79.

Children with ADHD Almost Always Have Other Disorders

A school population of seven-year-old children was clinically examined. The children were followed up two to four years later.

RESULTS

- 87 per cent of the children who were diagnosed as having ADHD had at least one additional disorder and 67 per cent had two additional disorders.

- The most common additional disorder in children with ADHD was oppositional defiant disorder.

- Development co-ordination disorder (below-average performance of daily activities needing motor co-ordination) and reading/writing disorder were, respectively, the second and third most common additional disorders in children with ADHD.

COMMENT

ADHD in isolation from other disorders is the exception, not the rule: this study points out the need to look for additional disorders in children with ADHD. The percentage of children with both ADHD and additional disorders may be higher in a clinical population than in this study of the general population.

This study was conducted in Sweden; however, similar results have been reported in studies conducted in North America.

SOURCE

Kadesjo, B. & Gillberg, C. (2001). The comorbidity of ADHD in the general population of Swedish school-age children. *Journal of Child Psychology and Psychiatry and Allied Disciplines, 42(4)*, 487–492.

Parent's Personality and Children with ADHD

Children with ADHD are more likely to become aggressive and antisocial than children without ADHD. This study examined parental characteristics that could contribute to the development of antisocial behaviour in boys with ADHD.

RESULTS

The results indicated that ADHD boys with aggressive and antisocial behaviours were likely to have had:

- mothers who have had major depressive or marked anxiety symptoms in the past year
- fathers with a childhood history of ADHD who were less agreeable, more neurotic, and more likely to have had generalized anxiety disorder.

SOURCE

Nigg, J.T. (1998). Parent personality traits and psychopathology associated with antisocial behaviors in childhood attention-deficit hyperactivity disorder. *Journal of Child Psychology and Psychiatry, 29*, 145–159.

Parents' Psychopathology and Children with ADHD

More than half of the children diagnosed with ADHD also have external-izing disorders (i.e., disorders that include aggressive and antisocial behaviours), such as conduct disorders (CD) or oppositional defiant dis-orders (ODD). This study looked at internalizing disorders (anxiety and depression) in children with ADHD. It also examined the relationship of the children's disorders to parental disorders. Parent and child interviews were performed to assess the relationship.

RESULTS

As many as one-third to one-half of the children who met the diagnostic criteria for ADHD also met the criteria for a depressive or anxiety disor-der, on the basis of parent and child interviews.

In children with ADHD, internalizing disorders (anxiety and depression) were as common as externalizing disorders.

Parental psychopathology appears to be associated with child disorders in a specific manner among children with ADHD:

- Child internalizing disorders are strongly related to internalizing dis-orders in parents.

- Child externalizing disorders are strongly related to externalizing disorders in fathers but not mothers.

There is no evidence from this study that cross-categorical relationships exist:

- Parental externalizing disorders were not related to internalizing dis-orders in children.

- Parental internalizing disorders were not related to externalizing disorders in children.

- Depression and anxiety disorders in parents were related to anxiety disorders in children, but depression in parents was not related to depressive disorders in children.

COMMENT

Very often the presence of internalizing disorders is not recognized in children with externalizing disorders. This study suggests that children with externalizing disorders often have anxiety and depression; therefore, it is important to look for these symptoms when treating children with antisocial and aggressive behaviour.

SOURCE

Pfiffner, L., McBurnett, K., Lahey, B., Loeber, R., Green, S., Frick, P. & Rathouz, P. (1999). Association of parental psychopathology to the comorbid disorders of boys with attention deficit hyperactivity. *Journal of Consulting and Clinical Psychology, 67*, 881–893.

Preschool Children with ADHD

RESULTS

Children between the ages of three and five with ADHD:

- were more non-compliant, had more difficult and inappropriate behaviour, and were less socially skilled than children without the disorder, and

- showed more negative social behaviour in preschool settings and scored significantly lower on a test of pre-academic skills.

Parents of children with ADHD:

- showed more negative behaviour toward their children, felt greater stress and coped less well than parents of children without ADHD.

SOURCE

DuPaul, G.J., McGoey, K.E., Eckert, T.L. & VanBrankle, J. (2001). Preschool children with attention-deficit/hyperactivity disorder: Impairments in behavioral, social, and school functioning. *Journal of the American Academy of Child and Adolescent Psychiatry, 40(5)*, 508–515.

Sleep Patterns in Children with ADHD

Disrupted or shortened sleep has been associated with attention-deficit hyperactivity disorder, difficult early temperament and later childhood behaviour problems. This study looked at whether 38 boys with ADHD were more prone to changes in sleep patterns night-to-night by comparing nightly time of falling asleep, amount of sleep, number of awakenings per night and other measures of sleep quality. These results were compared to 64 other school-aged boys. Measurement was by actigraphy, which is activity-based monitoring by a wristwatch-like device.

RESULTS

- In general, over the five nights of study, the boys with ADHD had greater variation of sleep measures compared to the other boys.

- In particular, the boys with ADHD had significant changes in nightly sleep onset time, sleep duration and true sleep time (amount of sleep without being awake).

IMPLICATIONS

A recent study also found that teenagers with irregular sleep habits had more behavioural problems and poorer results in school.

Sleep could be very important in school-aged children with learning or behavioural problems. Sleep issues should be discussed in any assessment of children with such problems.

If sleep problems are suspected, a more thorough sleep study may be worthwhile, to look at sleep quantity and quality.

SOURCE

Gruber, R., Sadeh, A. & Raviv, A. (2000). A study of differences in sleep patterns between ADHD boys and those without ADHD. *Journal of the American Academy of Child and Adolescent Psychiatry, 39(4),* 495–501.

ADHD and Girls

Perhaps because many more boys than girls have ADHD, most studies of children with ADHD are of boys. This study examined girls who were diagnosed with ADHD. A matched sample of boys with ADHD from a previous study was selected for comparison.

RESULTS

- The two groups were very similar on many measures. However, most of the symptoms were more severe in girls than boys, with the exception of hyperactivity, which the teachers, but not the parents, reported to be more severe in boys.

- The girls and boys did not differ in their response to drugs (methylphenidate and dextroamphetamine). Both responded well to the medications.

SOURCE

Sharp, W.S., Walter, J.M., Marsh, W.L., Ritchie, G.F., Hamburger, S.D. & Castellanos, F.X. (1999). ADHD in girls: Clinical comparability of a research sample. *Journal of the American Academy of Child and Adolescent Psychiatry, 38,* 40–47.

Adolescent Females with ADHD

This study compared adolescent females with ADHD to those without ADHD and to males with ADHD.

RESULTS

Adolescent females with ADHD:

- had more depression, anxiety, low self-esteem and stress

- commonly reported past suicidal ideas

- showed no difference from the other groups in amount of drug use.

The results also revealed that:

- Teachers and parents reported similar observations about the degree of accompanying problems in adolescent females with ADHD.

- Females and males with ADHD showed similar cognitive impairment but females with ADHD showed greater psychological impairment. This implies that special attention should be paid to both emotional and intellectual difficulties in females with ADHD.

COMMENT

Female adolescents with ADHD may be more vulnerable to psychological problems than their male counterparts. People in close contact with youth, including teachers, parents and therapists, should address not only the ADHD symptoms but also the many possible mental health problems that may accompany it.

SOURCE

Rucklidge, J.J. & Tannock, R. (2001). Psychiatric, psychosocial, and cognitive functioning of female adolescents with ADHD. *Journal of the American Academy of Child and Adolescent Psychiatry, 40(5),* 530–540.

Influence of Gender on ADHD

Girls with ADHD have many of the same symptoms, comorbid disorders, social dysfunction and cognitive impairments as boys with ADHD. However, more boys than girls have ADHD: estimates are 10 boys for every girl in clinic-referred cases and three boys for every girl among community-referred cases.

This study compared boys and girls with and without ADHD in different areas of functioning to discover more about the differences between girls and boys with ADHD.

RESULTS

Compared to boys with ADHD, girls with ADHD are:

- more likely to have the primarily inattentive type of ADHD
- less likely to have an associated learning disability in reading or mathematics
- less likely to have problems in school
- more likely to have substance use disorders
- less likely to have disruptive behaviour disorders (conduct disorder, oppositional defiant disorder)
- less likely to have major depression
- less likely to receive pharmacotherapy and psychotherapy
- more likely to have panic disorder.

COMMENT

The typical age of onset for ADHD differs by at least 10 years from that of substance use disorders. It was surprising, therefore, to find that girls with ADHD were more likely to have substance use problems. As a result, girls with ADHD should receive prevention programs for substance use problems as soon as ADHD is diagnosed.

The authors point out that disruptive behaviour is less common in girls with ADHD than in boys. This may explain the high rate of clinic referrals of boys compared to girls, as disruptive behaviour is generally the reason for referral to a clinic. This may also explain the different ratios of boys to girls in clinic-referred cases (10 to one) and non-clinic referrals (three to one).

SOURCE

Biederman, J., Mick, E., Faraone, S.V., Braaten, E., Doyle, A., Spencer, T., Wilens, T.E., Frazier, E. & Johnson, M.A. (2002). Influence of gender on attention deficit hyperactivity disorder in children referred to a psychiatric clinic. *American Journal of Psychiatry, 159(1)*, 36–42.

How Much Do Teachers Know about ADHD?

Attention-deficit hyperactivity disorder (ADHD) is the most common disorder among school-aged children, affecting approximately three to five per cent of them. If teachers are educated about the cause and treatment of ADHD, they can manage children with ADHD better in the classroom and collaborate with physicians in assessment and treatment. This study aimed to assess teachers' attitudes, training and knowledge about ADHD.

Forty-four teachers completed a 27-item knowledge test both before and after receiving an ADHD curriculum developed by the U.S. national organization Children and Adults with Attention Deficit Disorders (CHADD). The CHADD Educators' Inservice program gives teachers information on ADHD diagnosis, treatment and classroom management strategies. It also helps teachers who work with students with ADHD to become more directly involved with physicians.

RESULTS

- Although teachers scored fairly well on the pretest of ADHD knowledge, results of the ADHD knowledge test at pre-intervention indicated that:
  - 41 per cent of the teachers thought that poor parenting could cause ADHD.
  - 41 per cent of the teachers thought that sugar or food additives could cause ADHD.
  - 64 per cent thought that methylphenidate (Ritalin) should be used only as a last resort.
- Post-intervention, the percentages of teachers holding these beliefs were 7 per cent, 5 per cent and 34 per cent, respectively.

COMMENT

The teachers' knowledge gaps concerning ADHD were similar to those reported in other studies. Teachers who learn about ADHD and are more directly involved with physicians who treat this disorder may find they are more effective and experience less stress in educating students with ADHD.

SOURCE

Barbaresi, W.J. & Olsen, R.D. (1998). An ADHD educational intervention for elementary schoolteachers: A pilot study. *Developmental and Behavioral Pediatrics, 19,* 94–100.

Treatment

What Does and Does Not Work for Children with ADHD?

RESULTS

In this critical review of treatments for children with ADHD, the authors conclude that:

- Medications such as Ritalin (methylphenidate):
  - have significant benefits in many areas, including classroom performance
  - have not proven effective in improving long-term academic achievement
  - have no effect on whether the children are liked more or less by their peers
  - have not been shown to improve long-term prognosis.
- Training parents in behavioural methods (rewarding good behaviour and ignoring or punishing difficult behaviour) produces good results.
- Behavioural interventions in classroom settings have proven effective.
- Cognitive-behavioural therapies (which include verbal self-instructions, problem solving skills, self-monitoring and other therapies aimed at

improving attention and impulse control) do not lead to positive results in behaviour or academic performance.

• Because of poor attention span and lack of impulse control, children with ADHD are unable to learn and employ the cognitive-behavioural techniques and monitor their own behaviour.

COMMENT

It is suggested that multimodal treatments may be the most cost-effective treatment for children with ADHD. Multimodal treatment involves a combination of small doses of stimulant medication (e.g., Ritalin) with behavioural treatments.

SOURCE

Pelham, Jr., W.E., Wheeler, T. & Chronis, A. (1998). Empirically supported psychosocial treatments for attention deficit hyperactivity disorder. *Journal of Clinical Child Psychology, 27,* 190–205.

What Is the Most Effective Treatment for Children with ADHD?

Attention-deficit hyperactivity disorder (ADHD) is the most-diagnosed behaviour disorder in North America. About three to five per cent of school-aged children in North America meet the diagnostic criteria for ADHD.

Current strategies for managing ADHD in children include:

• medication to reduce the frequency and intensity of problematic behaviours and allow the child to have better self-control and attention to tasks

• parent and teacher education about ADHD to support realistic expectations of the child, provide simple strategies to modify environments to help reduce behaviour problems and teach effective behaviour-management skills

• psychological therapy to teach the child self-control and self-monitoring skills.

There is concern that in North America ADHD may be overdiagnosed and psychostimulants (e.g., Ritalin) to treat it overprescribed. ADHD is both diagnosed and treated by prescription medication less frequently in other parts of the world, such as Europe and Australia.

Some concerns around the prescription of psychostimulants for ADHD are:

- safety of medication for individual patients and possible adverse effects

- potential for illicit use and misuse of psychostimulants

- economic impact of increasing prescriptions

- relative effectiveness and safety of non-drug interventions.

This paper examined three treatment strategies for ADHD for relative effectiveness:

- medication only

- behavioural therapies

- a combination of medication and behavioural therapy.

An extensive literature review led to 26 studies that met the criteria of the researchers. Diagnoses of ADHD were based on parents' and teachers' completed questionnaires on the children's behaviour (Hyperactivity Index of Conners' Teacher Rating Scale and Conners' Parent Rating Scale are two widely used measures). The three treatment conditions were tested against either a no-treatment or a placebo condition. In the majority of the studies (22 of 26), children were randomly assigned these conditions.

RESULTS

- Medication-only therapy was effective in reducing the symptoms of ADHD.

- Behavioural therapies used alone appeared to be ineffective; however, only two studies were analysed in this category, involving small samples and poor methodological quality.

- Combination therapy was:

  - more effective than placebo or no treatment, in parent but not teacher ratings

  - not more effective than drug therapy alone

  - more effective than behavioural treatments alone based on parent but not teacher ratings.

COMMENT

As drug therapy alone was found to be beneficial, it was expected that combination therapy would be at least as effective as drug therapy alone. However, the results of this study suggest that medical therapy is more effective than behavioural therapy alone or in combination. That being said, only three studies examined the effectiveness of combined medication and behaviour therapies—and they relied on small samples and mixed methodological quality. Until more quality research is available, it is impossible to make conclusions about the relative effectiveness of these types of therapies.

The authors suggest that medication may be more effective in reducing the main symptoms of ADHD, while behavioural therapies may be more effective in resolving other aspects of ADHD, such as conflict with peers and poor academic performance. However, because most studies use behavioural ratings to measure the effect of treatment, rather than measures such as direct client observation or measures of individual treatment, the effectiveness of therapy other than medication may be hard to assess.

The authors discuss other problems with evaluating the effects of behavioural treatments in controlled experimental studies. For example, children with ADHD present a different array of symptoms and problems to clinicians, parents, teachers and peers, which cannot be categorized in one group. Likewise, no standard form of behaviour therapy applies to all cases; treatment must be in tune with the individual needs and differences of the child. However, testing the effects of medication therapy lends itself well to controlled experimental studies.

SOURCE

Klassen, A., Miller, A., Raina, P., Lee, S.K. & Olsen, L. (1999). Attention-deficit hyperactivity disorder in children and youth: A quantitative systematic review of the efficacy of different management strategies. *Canadian Journal of Psychiatry, 44*, 1007–1016.

ADHD: Does Training Parents Help?

This study was designed to determine the effectiveness of training in improving parents' knowledge of ADHD and techniques for behaviour management. It was assumed that improvements in these areas would result in improved behaviour of the children with ADHD. The children in this study were also receiving appropriate medication for the disorder.

Parents attended six 90-minute group sessions. Sessions were held on a weekly basis. Parents were provided with factual knowledge of the disorder, taught behaviour management techniques and given the medications for their children.

RESULTS

- Parents' knowledge and understanding of ADHD improved.

- Parents' behaviour management skills improved.

- The behaviour of the children did not improve.

- The parents had a modest degree of stress reduction.

COMMENT

Most studies suggest that the best treatment for children with ADHD includes medication, working with the parents and special programming in the school. Consequently, it was surprising that parent training did not result in improvements in the children's behaviour. However, the fact that the parents experienced some reduction in their stress was a positive finding.

SOURCE

Weinberg, H.A. (1999). Parent training for Attention-Deficit Hyperactivity Disorder: Parental and child outcome. *Journal of Clinical Psychology, 55,* 907–913.

Treatment of ADHD in Adolescents with Substance Use and Conduct Disorders

Research has shown that:

- Among adolescents with substance use disorders (SUD) and conduct disorders (CD), 30 to 50 per cent also have ADHD.

- In young people with CD, comorbid (co-occurring) ADHD is associated with more severe CD and earlier onset of CD as well as substance dependence.

- Comorbid ADHD may increase the chance that both SUD and antisocial behaviours continue into adulthood.

This article outlined clinical principles to guide the evaluation and treatment of these difficult comorbid conditions. The following questions were addressed:

How is ADHD diagnosed in the presence of concurrent SUD and CD?

Clinicians are often concerned that observed attention deficits and hyperactivity problems may be substance induced, and thus, not ADHD.

One way to help diagnose ADHD is to determine the age of onset of the disorder. ADHD can usually be diagnosed before age seven, which is almost always before the onset of either SUD or CD.

Getting a clear history from parents, school reports and the client will help to determine if diagnostic criteria were met early in childhood and whether symptoms have been continuously present.

To safeguard against adolescents who over-report symptoms of ADHD to be prescribed psychostimulants (e.g., Ritalin):

• determine if there has been any previous abuse of medications; and

• pay attention to DSM-IV and dependence criteria to help distinguish between common "experimentation" and more serious drug or alcohol use.

How should clinicians treat ADHD in clients with comorbid ADHD, SUD and CD?

The authors point out the following:

• Treating adolescents with medications such as pemoline or bupropion, which are similar in effectiveness to psychostimulants but have a lower abuse potential, may prevent potential misuse of prescribed psychostimulants.

• Tricyclic antidepressants may have undesirable interactions when used with illicit substances.

How do clinicians integrate the treatment of ADHD, SUD and CD?

The authors recommend that:

• Cognitive-behavioural techniques, as well as a systemic family therapy approach, should be used to treat the SUD.

• Cautious and carefully monitored use of prescription medication for ADHD can begin once substance use is significantly reduced.

- Medication should only be given by a supervising adult and must be stored in a secure place.

SOURCE

Riggs, P.D. (1998). Clinical approach to treatment of ADHD in adolescents with substance use disorders and conduct disorder. *Journal of the American Academy of Child and Adolescent Psychiatry, 37,* 331–332.

Psychoeducational Interventions for Children with ADHD

School-based interventions for children with ADHD can improve both academic performance and behaviour. The following are some interventions that have proven helpful.

Interventions for elementary students

Consequence-based strategies

Token reinforcements

- These work well, because tokens give immediate and frequent reinforcements following the desired behaviour.

- The rewards must be important to the child.

- It is useful to have a menu of reinforcers available that the child can choose from at the beginning of the day or class period.

Mild form of punishment (loss of privileges)

- Positive reinforcements are not always enough to modify behaviour.

- In response to major undesirable behaviours, the child loses a privilege or tokens earned.

Strategies aimed at preventing antisocial behaviour

Making choices

- making fewer demands

- making tasks more stimulating

- giving students choices in their academic work.

Peer tutoring

- Two students work together on an academic activity, with one student helping and instructing the other.

Computer-assisted instruction

- A highly appealing interactive format that stimulates multiple sensory modalities.

Interventions for secondary school students

Note-taking

- Note-taking is an important skill to acquire in secondary school, especially in content-area courses (e.g., history).

- Students are given a notebook and the teacher shows why some information is considered main-topic material and why other information is considered supporting-detail material.

Peer coaching

- The student with ADHD works with a coach who is either a teacher or a peer who does not have ADHD.

School-home notes

- Communication between school and home is critical to monitor the student's ongoing academic and behavioural performance.

- The exchange of daily or weekly notes enables school-home communication.

Contingency contracting

- The teacher and student negotiate an agreement in which they specify the desired behavioural outcome, goal and reward.

Progress monitoring

To determine the effectiveness of the intervention, progress should be monitored in an objective and measurable fashion.

Source

Hoffman, J.B. & DuPaul, G.J. (2000). Psychoeducational interventions for children and adolescents with attention-deficit/hyperactivity disorder. *Child and Adolescent Psychiatric Clinics of North America, 9(3),* 647–661.

Another Medication for ADHD

Methylphenidate (Ritalin) is a stimulant commonly used to treat ADHD, with good results. In one study, methylphenidate normalized classroom behaviour in 78 per cent of children treated. However, it has many disadvantages:

- Its side-effects include insomnia and loss of appetite.
- Its effects last only three to four hours.
- It has the potential for misuse and dependence.

In this study, buspirone (an anti-anxiety drug) was given to 12 children with ADHD. The dose was 0.5 milligrams per kilogram of body weight. The dose ranged between 15 to 30 milligrams given in two doses a day and was administered for six weeks.

RESULTS

- Children improved in the areas of hyperactivity, impulsivity, inattention and disruptive behaviour.
- The only side-effect reported was slight dizziness.

COMMENT

Many parents object to Ritalin because of its side-effects and potential for misuse; buspirone provides a practical alternative.

SOURCE

Malhotra, S. & Santosh, P.J. (1998). An open clinical trial of buspirone in children with attention-deficit/hyperactivity disorder. *Journal of the American Academy of Child and Adolescent Psychiatry, 37,* 364–371.

Chapter 5
Juvenile Offenders

Juvenile Offenders

Youth between ages 12 and 18 who have been charged with a criminal offence. Included are homicidal youth, sexual offenders and property offenders.

Characteristics and Related Issues

What Happens to Girls with Antisocial Behaviour?

Until recently, research on adult outcomes of antisocial behaviour in youth focused primarily on males. This may have stemmed, in part, from widespread beliefs that antisocial behaviour in females was rare and a stage they would "grow out of." More recent research shows that antisocial behaviour in females is neither rare nor temporary.

Study 1

This was a review of previous studies of adult outcomes of adolescent girls with antisocial behaviour problems.

RESULTS

- Conduct disorder is the second most common diagnosis in adolescent girls.

- 7.5 per cent to 9.5 per cent of girls meet the criteria for conduct disorder, compared to 8.6 per cent to 12.2 per cent of boys.

- Self-reports of antisocial behaviour indicate that girls report the same patterns of antisocial behaviour as boys, with the exception of sexual assault.

- Unlike boys, whose antisocial behaviour in adolescence is likely to result in criminal behaviour in adulthood, girls may manifest ongoing antisocial behaviour in different ways in adulthood.

- Some adolescent girls begin their antisocial behaviour during early adolescence and continue to commit offences with increasing severity and frequency into adulthood. Others start with norm violation (e.g., coming home late and missing school) and continue into adulthood with less serious criminal offences (e.g., substance use) and continued contact with peers who engage in antisocial behaviours.

- As adults, girls with antisocial behaviour problems manifest

    - increased mortality rates

    - 10- to 40-fold increase in criminality rates (an estimated 25 per cent to 50 per cent engage in adult criminal behaviour)

    - substantial rates of mental illness

- dysfunctional and often violent relationships

- high rates of multiple-service use.

COMMENT

Although the results of this review are provocative, there were some concerns about the past research:

• Data was mostly on white females; therefore, results may not generalize to other racial groups.

• Many of the studies did not use a control group for comparison purposes.

• Outcome measures and definitions of antisocial behaviour were not uniform.

Despite the shortcomings of past research, it is clear that antisocial behaviour in adolescent girls has important long-term individual and social consequences. This area warrants further research using improved research methods.

SOURCE

Pajer, K.A. (1998). What happens to "bad" girls?: A review of the adult outcomes of antisocial adolescents. *American Journal of Psychiatry, 155,* 862–870.

Study 2

This study examined the physical health outcomes of adolescent girls with behaviour problems. Girls were first examined at age 15 and then followed up at 21. In all, 459 girls were evaluated. They were grouped as having:

• no disorder

• conduct disorder

• depressive or anxiety disorder.

Some girls had a combination of disorders; however, the researchers were able to analyse the disorders in isolation by using statistical methods.

At age 21, general health, substance dependence and reproductive health were assessed. To assess general health, the young women completed a standard medical intake questionnaire indicating which of 13 medical problems they had experienced since age 15. The Diagnostic Interview

Schedule was used to assess substance dependence. Questions about reproductive health were drawn from the British National Survey of Sexual Attitudes and Lifestyles.

RESULTS

- Compared with the other groups, girls with conduct disorder grew up to have:
  - more medical problems (according to the standard medical intake completed at age 21)
  - poorer self-reported overall health
  - lower body weight
  - more substance use problems
  - greater risk for reproductive health problems.
- Adolescent depression-only predicted tobacco dependence in adulthood and more medical problems.
- Adolescent anxiety-only predicted more medical problems.

COMMENT

The results suggest a broad link between conduct disorder in adolescent girls and poor physical health in young adulthood. However, the links between anxiety or depression and physical health were not as broad.

While poor physical health on its own is a problem, it is worse when combined with the other long-term difficulties associated with conduct disorder in young women (i.e., economic disadvantage, young motherhood, abusive relationships). To prevent the accumulation of psychological, socio-economic and physical health problems, the authors stress the importance of intensive early intervention.

SOURCE

Bardone, A.M., Moffitt, T.E., Caspi, A., Dickson, N., Stanton, W.R. & Silva, P.A. (1998). Adult physical health outcomes of adolescent girls with conduct disorder, depression, and anxiety. *Journal of the American Academy of Child and Adolescent Psychiatry, 37*, 594–601.

Post-Traumatic Stress Disorder (PTSD) in Female Juvenile Offenders

Although many studies indicate the presence of psychopathology (abnormal, maladaptive behaviour or thoughts) in male juvenile offenders, there are relatively few such studies of female offenders. This study examines the presence of post-traumatic stress disorder (PTSD) in female juvenile offenders and its effect on social and emotional adjustment. It is the first study to examine the incidence of PTSD in incarcerated female offenders.

Diagnostic criteria for PTSD include:

- a history of exposure to a "traumatic event"
- symptoms such as high levels of anxiety, depression, aggression, various physical complaints and withdrawal.

RESULTS

Trauma

- 70 per cent of the young women had been exposed to some form of trauma.
- 74 per cent reported being hurt or in danger of being hurt.
- 76 per cent reported witnessing someone being severely injured or killed.
- 60 per cent reported being raped or in danger of being raped.

Socio-emotional adjustment

- The young women with PTSD showed higher levels of distress (which relates to anxiety, depression and low self-esteem) and lower levels of self-restraint.

PTSD

- 65.3 per cent of the young women had symptoms of PTSD at some time in their lives.
- 48.9 per cent were experiencing the symptoms of PTSD at the time of the study.

COMMENT

Female juvenile offenders are 50 per cent more likely to have PTSD than male juvenile offenders. Females are also more likely than males to develop symptoms of PTSD after a traumatic incident. The explanation may be that females are more likely to be victims of violence than witnesses, and people who are victims of violence are more likely to experience mental health problems than those who only witness violence.

The clinical implications are that:

• The presence of PTSD may make rehabilitative efforts less effective; for example, PTSD may increase impulsivity.

• All female offenders should be examined for the symptoms of PTSD. Often they are referred for attention problems when PTSD is the problem.

SOURCE

Cauffman, E., Feldman, S.S., Waterman, J. & Steiner, H. (1998). Post-traumatic stress disorder among female juvenile offenders. *Journal of the American Academy of Child and Adolescent Psychiatry, 37,* 1209–1216.

Hyperactive Boys and Criminality

Past studies have shown that children who are hyperactive are more likely to get involved in criminal behaviour during adolescence than other children. In this study, boys who were diagnosed as hyperactive between the ages of six and 12 were followed up to age 23.

RESULTS

The results of this follow-up suggest that boys who are hyperactive are more likely to:

• commit offences that will lead to arrest and incarceration in adulthood

• be arrested in adulthood if they are arrested during adolescence

• continue offending in adulthood if arrested in the early years of adolescence (as opposed to the later years)

• have higher rates of recidivism in adulthood if their first arrest occurs before age 15

- continue offending into adulthood if they have multiple arrests during adolescence.

COMMENT

The authors found that a single juvenile arrest for a violent offence is not a good predictor of adult arrest for violent offences; therefore, "one strike and you are out" is not a good policy. In summary, boys diagnosed as hyperactive are at greatest risk to continue offending into adulthood if they:

- offend before the age of 15,

- commit more than one offence, and

- have multiple arrests.

SOURCE

Satterfield, J.H. & Schell, A. (1997). A prospective study of hyperactive boys with conduct problems and normal boys: Adolescent and adult criminality. *Journal of the American Academy of Child and Adolescent Psychiatry, 36*, 1726–1735.

Psychiatric Disorders in Juvenile Offenders

Fifty adolescents (45 boys and five girls) from a juvenile detention centre were interviewed and completed the Diagnostic Interview Schedule for Children. Their mean age was 15.4.

RESULTS

- 24 per cent did not meet the criteria for any diagnosis.

- Of the 76 per cent who did meet criteria for diagnosis, many of the young people met the criteria for more than one diagnosis:

  - 60 per cent met the criteria for conduct disorder.

  - 24 per cent met the criteria for oppositional defiant disorder.

  - 18 per cent met the criteria for ADHD.

  - 42 per cent met the criteria for affective disorder.

- Alcohol dependence was found in 28 per cent of the young offenders and marijuana dependence in 46 per cent.

COMMENT

Many studies have shown that juvenile offenders often have psychiatric and neurological disorders, yet most detention centres do not screen them for these disorders. This study indicates that many juvenile offenders have depression or mania or both, and need treatment. Such treatment could alter the future of these young people, possibly helping to reduce their chances of reoffending.

SOURCE

Pliszka, S.R., Sherman, J.O., Barrow, M.V. & Irick, S. (2000). Affective disorder in juvenile offenders: A preliminary study. *American Journal of Psychiatry, 157*, 130–132.

Personality Traits and Recidivism in Juvenile Offenders

In the treatment of juvenile offenders, the high rate of recidivism remains a serious problem. One recent study reported that 69 per cent of juvenile offenders on parole were rearrested for serious crimes within six years of release. Meanwhile, the number of youth involved in violent crime keeps rising—youth arrested for violent crimes increased by 64 per cent between 1987 and 1995.

This study examined the relationship between criminal behaviour, recidivism and two personality traits: distress and restraint. In all, 481 incarcerated juvenile offenders completed questionnaires assessing distress and restraint as personality characteristics. Distress and restraint are two personality traits measured by the Weinberger Adjustment Inventory, which has 62 items in total. According to the measure, distress relates to anxiety, depression and low self-esteem; restraint relates to impulsivity, aggression, lack of a sense of responsibility and the inability to be considerate of others.

RESULTS

- Juvenile offenders who showed low levels of restraint:
  - had more previous offences
  - received more institutional punishments
  - were more likely to have been rearrested.

- Juvenile offenders who showed high levels of distress:

  - were more likely to have committed crimes both against people and against property

  - were unlikely to have received institutional punishments or lengthy incarceration.

- Those who showed low levels of both distress and restraint were the most likely to be rearrested.

COMMENT

Other studies have shown that anxiety and depression act as protective factors against the development of antisocial behaviour. Therefore, it was surprising to find that the young people in this study who had high levels of anxiety and depression were more likely to have committed crimes against people and property. The study's authors suggest that there are two types of violent behaviours—predatory (planned for personal gain) and affective (resulting from an emotional state)—to explain these findings. Thus, affective disturbance (e.g., anxiety, depression) may be an additional pathway to criminal antisocial behaviour.

SOURCE

Steiner, H., Cauffman, E. & Duxbury, E. (1999). Personality traits in juvenile delinquents: Relation to criminal behavior and recidivism. *Journal of the American Academy of Child and Adolescent Psychiatry, 38*, 256–262.

Recidivism in Juvenile Sexual Offenders

This study included 170 first-time sexual offenders (of which three were female).

RESULTS

These juvenile sexual offenders had the following characteristics:

- 45.7 per cent had also committed non-sexual offences.

- 61 per cent molested only one victim.

- Most had molested female victims; only 25.9 per cent selected male victims.

- Most selected family members or acquaintances as victims. In 69.1 per cent of the cases, the victim was a relative; in only 13.5 per cent the victim was a stranger.

- 66 per cent molested children under eight years old.

- 44 per cent had experienced sexual or physical abuse or both. The mean age at the time of abuse was eight.

Factors related to recidivism

Molestation of multiple victims rather than one victim increased the chances of committing future sexual offences. However, those who molested one victim (as opposed to multiple victims) were more likely to commit non-sexual offences.

Parents' divorce or separation was associated with recidivism, but this was more strongly associated with non-sexual recidivism.

Those who had a history of child sexual abuse as victims were more likely to reoffend sexually.

COMMENT

Treatment programs should address the factors that contribute to *all* criminal behaviours and their persistence, not just sexual offending.

Identification of characteristics associated with recidivism (e.g., divorce/separation of parents, history of child sexual abuse) may help clinicians identify issues to highlight as treatment goals and whom to involve in treatment.

Treatment programs should encourage family involvement: adequate family support helps prevent recidivism in young offenders.

SOURCE

Rasmussen, L.A. (1999). Factors related to recidivism among juvenile sexual offenders. *Sexual Abuse: A Journal of Research and Treatment, 11*, 69–85.

Divorce, Remarriage and Antisocial Behaviour

This study examined the impact of divorce and remarriage on the development of antisocial behaviour in a group of 427 boys. The boys were from low-income families. They were followed from age six to between ages 10 and 15. At the start of the study, all families were intact; at the end, 334 of the families remained intact. The boys were grouped according to whether they experienced divorce or remarriage in their family and when it occurred.

RESULTS

- Boys who experienced the *remarriage* of parents between ages 12 and 15 experienced more problems than boys whose families remained intact. They:

    - engaged in violent activities, such as gang fights and hurting innocent people, and antisocial activities, such as stealing

    - engaged in much more antisocial activity than boys from intact families until age 14; however, by age 15, their levels of antisocial behaviour decreased to the same level as that of other boys

    - reported being supervised less and perceived their relationship with their parents to be less supportive and expressive than other boys.

COMMENT

Responding to the question of why this age group of boys who experienced remarriage did worse than other groups, the authors point out the following:

- These boys experienced two transitions, divorce and remarriage, instead of just one or none.

- Transition occurred at an age when delinquency typically increases and parent-child relationships are often strained.

- Custodial parents who remarried may have been parenting less effectively because of the demands of being involved in a new relationship.

Interestingly, the boys whose parents divorced but did not remarry did not differ significantly from those whose families remained intact.

SOURCE

Pagani, L., Tremblay, R.E., Vitaro, F., Kerr, M. & McDuff, P. (1998). The impact of family transition on the development of delinquency in adolescent boys: A 9-year longitudinal study. *Journal of Child Psychology and Psychiatry, 39*, 489–499.

Causes and Contributing Factors

Why Boys Join Gangs

The growth of the gang phenomenon is an increasing concern. It is estimated that 650,000 youths in the United States are members of gangs. The violence associated with gang membership not only harms the victims but also exposes gang members to risk of injury, incarceration and death. If we can learn more about what influences young boys to join gangs, then we can decrease both juvenile crime rates and risk of harm to gang members.

Two major models try to explain why boys enter gangs:

- One model suggests that boys who already engage in antisocial behaviour enter gangs to join with people like themselves.

- The other model suggests boys enter gangs for self-esteem, power and protection. According to this model, gang membership encourages antisocial behaviour.

Both theories have some merit in explaining why young people join gangs and how antisocial behaviour may be escalated through gang membership.

This article is based on data collected from the six-year longitudinal Pittsburgh Youth Study (PYS). In this study, the researchers tried to replicate research findings that future gang membership can be predicted both by the individual's antisocial behaviour before gang entry and by family and neighbourhood characteristics. The participants were 375 boys (204 African-American and 143 white males) from the PYS. The boys were in Grade 7 of an urban public school system at the start of the study.

RESULTS

- 95 boys reported entering a gang either before or after the study began.

- 62 boys reported entry into "serious" gangs (gangs that engage in fighting, drug sales, stealing or homicide).

- By age 19, 8 per cent of the white boys and 34 per cent of the African-American boys had entered gangs.

To examine potential predictors of serious gang entry, information was compiled on 183 African-American boys whose gang entry occurred during the data collection. (Because only two white boys had entered a serious gang, the study is limited to predicting gang entry of African-American boys.)

- 25 of the 183 African-American boys reported entering a serious gang.

- Factors such as prior behaviour/conduct problems, association with peers with antisocial behaviour problems, low family income and low levels of parental supervision were found to be predictors of gang entry. However, these findings were dependent on age:

  - The association between initial behaviour problems and entry into a serious gang was weakened as age increased.

  - Friendships with aggressive peers were related to serious gang entry only during early adolescence.

  - Higher family income seemed to protect youth from gang entry in late adolescence, but it was associated with higher risk of serious gang entry during early adolescence.

  - Less parental supervision increased the risk of serious gang entry during early adolescence, but was associated with lower risk in late adolescence.

COMMENT

In early adolescence, friendships with peers engaged in antisocial behaviours may lead to gang membership, but in general, gang entry may reflect a tendency for boys with antisocial behaviour problems to associate with one another.

Due to limited data, the authors could not explain the relationship between family income and age.

In early adolescence, boys with conduct problems who receive low parental supervision may be the first to join gangs, whereas boys who join gangs in late adolescence may have been deterred by greater parental supervision in early adolescence.

SOURCE

Lahey, B.B., Gordon, R.A., Loeber, R., Stouthamer-Loeber, M. & Farrington, D.P. (1999). Boys who join gangs: A prospective study of predictors of first gang entry. *Journal of Abnormal Child Psychology, 27*, 261–276.

Early Onset of Antisocial Behaviour May Be Genetically Determined

Early onset of antisocial behaviour may be the single best predictor of severity and persistence of antisocial behaviour in adulthood. Antisocial behaviour that starts in adolescence is supposed to be transitory (not permanent). Thus, there are two types of people with antisocial behaviour problems: those who begin antisocial behaviour early and those who start antisocial behaviour during adolescence.

This study aimed to determine the reasons for the differences between the two groups and test the hypothesis that there is greater genetic influence in early onset of antisocial behaviour than in late onset.

The study included twin boys, 63 identical and 33 fraternal twins, between the ages of 10 and 12, with a history of antisocial behaviour. The boys were divided into three groups:

- early onset, where antisocial behaviour started before age 12
- late onset, where antisocial behaviour started after age 12
- a control group, without antisocial behaviour problems.

RESULTS

- The boys whose antisocial behaviour started early differed from both other groups in that they had:
  - lower verbal and spatial memory functioning
  - more psychological and emotional problems related to inhibition
  - earlier and more persistent association with peers who had antisocial behaviours

- more cases of ADHD and oppositional defiant disorder

- higher scores on an impulsivity scale.

• The analysis of twins indicated that the risk of early onset was sub-
stantially greater for co-twins in monozygotic (identical) pairs (55
per cent concordant) than for co-twins in dizygotic (fraternal) pairs (29
per cent concordant) in which one boy started early.

• There was greater genetic influence for antisocial behaviour among the
early-onset group compared to the late-onset group:

  - The early starters had significantly more second-degree relatives
    with antisocial behaviour or conduct disorder in adulthood than did
    the control group.

  - The early starters had significantly more second-degree relatives
    with antisocial personality disorder (but not conduct disorder) than
    did the late starters.

CONCLUSION

This study gives evidence that there is a greater genetic influence in determining early onset of antisocial behaviour than late onset.

SOURCE

Taylor, J., Lacono, W.G., & McGue., M. (2000). Evidence for a genetic etiology of early-onset delinquency. *Journal of Abnormal Psychology, 109(4),*
634–643.

Family Interaction and Juvenile Offending

Various family interaction patterns have been linked to different forms of
adolescent antisocial behaviour, including delinquent offending. This
ongoing longitudinal study asked whether certain family interventions,
such as physical punishment, communication, supervision, positive parenting and child-parent relationships, remain stable. The study involved
boys from age six to 18 and their caretakers.

RESULTS

Physical punishment

• Level of physical punishment decreased over time.

- African-American and single-parent households reported more physical punishment than white or two-parent households.
- Boys who received higher levels of physical punishment engaged in more serious forms of antisocial behaviour.

Communication

- Level of communication got only slightly worse over time.
- Boys who came from single-parent households and those who were born to young mothers reported higher rates of poor communication than those from two-parent households and those born to older mothers.
- Boys who engaged in more serious forms of antisocial behaviour reported higher rates of poor communication.

Supervision

- Level of supervision decreased with age.
- African-American and single-parent households gave less supervision compared to white and two-parent households.
- Boys who committed more serious delinquency reported having less supervision.

Positive parenting

This relates to parents giving the child praise or approval for acts that meet with their favour.

- Level of positive parenting decreased after age 10.
- Boys from single-parent and white households received less positive parenting than those in two-parent and African-American households.

Relationship with primary caretaker

- Relationship improved with age for young boys, then worsened during adolescent years and levelled off in later years.
- Poor relationships between boys and their caretakers were more pronounced in single-parent households than in two-parent households.

COMMENT

This study should help identify categories of parents who can benefit from parent training programs to improve family interactions known to be associated with antisocial behaviour.

SOURCE

Loeber, R., Drinkwater, M., Yanming, Y., Stewart, A.J., Schmidt, L.C. & Crawford, A. (2000). Stability of family interaction from ages 6 to 18. *Journal of Abnormal Child Psychology, 28*, 353–369.

Disrupted Families and Antisocial Behaviour

Increases in antisocial behaviour in society rose simultaneously with increases in divorce rates. This has caused speculation about the connection between family breakdown and antisocial behaviour. Previous research reported that the risk of antisocial behaviour doubled for children who experienced parents' divorce or separation compared to those from intact families. This longitudinal study looked at a group of boys living in South London.

RESULTS

- Disruptions caused by disharmony were associated with higher rates of antisocial behaviour than were disruptions caused by death.

- Antisocial behaviour rates among boys from intact but high-conflict families were similar to the rates among boys from disrupted families.

- Antisocial behaviour rates of boys with single mothers whose fathers had died were lower than the rates of antisocial behaviour among boys in intact, low-conflict families.

- Antisocial behaviour rates of boys who were not with their mothers were very high, partly because the absence of the mother often led to several parental transitions.

- Family disruptions in infancy (under age five) or adolescence (age 10 to 14) were more damaging than family disruptions in childhood (age five to nine).

COMMENT

Although the results of this study indicated that the loss of a mother was more disruptive than the loss of a father, the authors point out that this may no longer be true. Fathers are more involved in the home and family now than when this study was conducted 40 years ago.

SOURCE

Juby, H. & Farrington, D.P. (2001). Disentangling the link between disrupted families and delinquency. *British Journal of Criminology, 41(1)*, 22–40.

Parental Support and Control and Antisocial Behaviour

This study analysed the impact of two concepts connected with prevention of antisocial behaviour: parental control and parental support. Previous research in this area found that:

- Emerging theory in criminology emphasizes how attempts at too much parental control can be counterproductive.

- Research in social psychology gives evidence that perceptions of social support have positive effects.

RESULTS

- This study found that, as distinct individual measures, the effects of parental control and support were modest. However, the effect of "parental efficacy"—a combination of control and support—appeared to be capable of limiting involvement in antisocial behaviour initially, and reducing it over a two-year period both in younger and in older youth.

- Parental efficacy is shown when parents build attachments (warm, caring relationships), set rules, monitor behaviour and spend time with their children. This form of parenting enhances a child's prosocial development and insulates against negative influences.

- Within families, individual youths appear to receive varying levels of attachment, supervision and rules. These variations account for differences in antisocial behaviour.

- Parental support is positively related to child-parent attachment, which is seen as an indirect control on antisocial behaviour. This is particularly important during adolescence—for poorly attached children, deviant peer groups are often a great attraction.

SOURCE

Wright, J.P. & Cullen, F.T. (2001). Parental efficacy and delinquent behavior: Do control and support matter? *Criminology, 39(3),* 677–705.

Adolescent Sex Offender: Victim and Offender

Adolescents are responsible for about 20 per cent of rapes and 30 to 50 per cent of cases of child sexual abuse. Past studies indicate that over 40 per cent of adolescent sexual offenders have a history of being sexually abused. The pathways to later offending are unclear. However, a history of sexual abuse may interact with feelings of social inadequacy, difficulties with intimacy and impulsiveness.

This study examined 74 adolescent male sex offenders referred or ordered for residential treatment. Histories of any past victimization were compared to their offences and victims.

RESULTS

- 92 per cent of these youth had a validated history of past sexual abuse.

- Those who were abused before age five were twice as likely to victimize someone younger than five.

- Youth who were abused by males themselves were twice as likely to sexually abuse a male.

- Boys subjected to anal intercourse were 15 times more likely to abuse their victims in this manner.

- Boys who were fondled were seven times more likely to fondle their victims.

COMMENT

A recent review of research did not indicate a clear relationship between prior sexual victimization and later offending. The authors in this study suggest that there may be a subgroup of adolescent sex offenders who re-enact their own abuse with others. However, it is hard to predict who will sexually abuse, and in what manner.

SOURCE

Veneziano, C., Veneziano, L. & LeGrand, S. (2000). A study of the relationship between characteristics of an offender's past victimization and subsequent offense. *Journal of Interpersonal Violence, 15(4),* 363–374.

Prevention

Leisure Activities and Antisocial Behaviour

The relationship of leisure activities to antisocial behaviour is not clear. Some studies indicate that leisure activities lower the chances of youth getting involved in antisocial behaviour, while other studies suggest the opposite. This study suggests that different results can be explained by the type of leisure activity: whether it is structured or unstructured.

Structured activities were defined as activities that happen at least once a week at a regular time, with others in the same age group and having an adult leader.

Unstructured activities are exemplified by youth recreation centres, where youth gather and are allowed to develop their own interests. Adults may be present but they do not direct or place demands on the youths' activity choices.

In this study, Grade 8 students and their parents answered questions related to the students' involvement in structured or unstructured activities during leisure time and their involvement in antisocial behaviour.

RESULTS

- Participation in structured activity is linked to low levels of antisocial behaviour.
- Unstructured leisure activity is associated with high levels of antisocial behaviour.

COMMENT

The authors conclude that youth should be offered structured leisure activities that are:

- aimed at skill building

- guided by rules
- led by a competent adult
- set up to follow a regular participation schedule.

Although this study was carried out in Sweden, similar results have been reported by studies conducted in North America.

SOURCE

Mahoney, J.L. & Stattin, H. (2000). Leisure activities and adolescent antisocial behavior: The role of structure and social context. *Journal of Adolescence, 23*, 113–127.

Treatment

Multi-systemic Treatment of Criminality and Violence

Adolescents who commit serious criminal and violent acts not only cause serious emotional and physical damage to victims, victims' families, the larger community and themselves, but they also place a large economic burden on society. They often have continued contact with the mental health and criminal justice systems well into adulthood.

Past research aimed at reducing recidivism among serious and violent juvenile offenders has been discouraging. Some treatments seem to be successful with relatively mild forms of antisocial behaviour (e.g., behavioural parent training, cognitive-behavioural therapy, functional family therapy). However, these interventions have been unsuccessful in treating serious antisocial behaviour.

More recently, multi-systemic therapy (MST) has received the most empirical support as an effective treatment for serious and violent criminal behaviour in adolescents. There is a growing consensus that effective treatments must have the capacity to intervene comprehensively—at individual, family, peer, school and possibly even neighbourhood levels. Programs such as "boot camps" have been ineffective because they take youth out of the real world environment that led to their criminal behaviour and to which they will eventually return. On the other hand, MST is effective because it is individualized, highly flexible and delivered in the youth's own environment (home, school, neighbourhood).

SOURCE

Borduin, C.M. (1998). Multisystemic treatment of criminality and violence in adolescents. *Journal of the American Academy of Child and Adolescent Psychiatry, 39,* 242–249.

Chapter 6
Abuse and Neglect

Abuse and Neglect

Abuse is the active physical, sexual or
emotional maltreatment of a child. Neglect
occurs when the physical and emotional
needs of the child are not met.

Characteristics and Related Issues

Five Years after Child Sexual Abuse

RESULTS

- This study found that sadness, depression, self-esteem and behaviour problems in a group of sexually abused children did not improve significantly over a period of approximately five years after disclosure.

- The five-year outcome of the sexually abused children in this study was extremely hard to predict. Nonetheless, some factors predicted outcome, such as further abuse, negative life events and family dysfunction.

COMMENT

The results in this study were in contrast to other studies that have reported improvement in overall behaviour over time following disclosure of abuse. The most surprising finding was that early intervention did not change the outcome in the five-year follow-up. However, the interventions varied considerably in duration, frequency, focus and quality. This study reinforces the importance of developing effective, well-researched treatment programs for sexually abused children.

The findings are yet another demonstration that the damaging effects of child sexual abuse persist over a long period of time. It is very difficult to predict which children will show improvement. However, this study did show that sexually abused children who are feeling sadness, depression or low self-esteem at the time of initial assessment are likely to have ongoing problems in these areas. As a result, this group may need extra therapeutic attention.

SOURCE

Tebbutt, J., Swanston, H., Oates, K.R. & O'Toole, B.I. (1997). Five years in a residential setting after child sexual abuse: Persisting dysfunction and problems of prediction. *Journal of the American Academy of Child and Adolescent Psychiatry, 36*, 330–339.

The Timing of Physical Abuse of Children

Past studies have shown that harsh physical punishment of children leads to behavioural and emotional problems during adolescence and later in life. This study examined the effect of the timing of physical abuse in two age groups: before age five and between ages six and nine. The objective was to determine if the consequences for the child differed according to the age period in which the physical maltreatment took place.

RESULTS

• Children who were physically abused before age five had more emotional and behavioural problems compared to children who were maltreated after five years old and children who were not maltreated.

• Children who were maltreated after age five were rated differently by mothers and teachers. Teachers and mothers both perceived the children as having behaviour problems. However, the mothers saw the children becoming less difficult over time, while the teachers saw the children becoming more difficult over time.

COMMENT

This study, like others, shows the harmful effects of physical abuse of children. In spite of overwhelming evidence, many parents continue to use physical punishment to discipline children. Teachers and mental health workers must continue to help parents in learning better, more effective ways of disciplining children.

SOURCE

Keiley, M.L., Howe, T.R., Dodge, K.A., Bates, J.E. & Petit, G.S. (2001). The timing of child physical maltreatment: A cross-domain growth analysis of impact on adolescent externalizing and internalizing problems. *Development and Psychopathology, 13(4),* 891–912.

Effects of Childhood Maltreatment on Adolescence

This study examined the connection between childhood maltreatment and clinically significant mental health problems in adolescence. Maltreatment included emotional, physical and sexual abuse as well as physical and emotional neglect.

RESULTS

- Childhood maltreatment is a significant risk factor for adolescent adjustments such as emotional distress, antisocial behaviour and dating violence.

- Female adolescents with histories of maltreatment reported emotional distress (anger, depression and anxiety), post-traumatic stress-related symptoms, and violent and non-violent antisocial acts.

- Male adolescents with histories of maltreatment reported fewer symptoms of emotional turmoil and antisocial behaviour than did females with histories of maltreatment.

- However, male adolescents with histories of maltreatment were significantly more likely to be abusive toward their dating partners.

COMMENT

In the clinical assessment of adolescents with emotional and antisocial behaviour problems, it is important to inquire about maltreatment. A history of maltreatment may explain many symptoms as well as indicate a line of treatment.

SOURCE

Wolfe, D.A., Scott, K., Wekerle, C. & Pittman, A.L. (2001). Child maltreatment: Risk of adjustment problems and dating violence in adolescence. *Journal of the American Academy of Child and Adolescent Psychiatry, 40(3)*, 282–289.

Maltreatment and Its Impact on Children

Maltreatment, which includes neglect and abuse of children, remains a serious problem in the United States. A recent report by the U.S. Department of Health and Human Services reported that nearly one in 24 children was the victim of maltreatment.

This study examined the effects of maltreatment on preschool children's emotional adjustment and social relationships. The study compared a group of maltreated children with a comparable group of non-maltreated children to see how they functioned in areas of peer play interaction, global social skills, peer assessments and teacher and parent ratings of behaviour.

RESULTS

Maltreated children

- had decreased peer play interaction
- had fewer social competencies
- had less self control
- were less liked by peers
- showed more internalizing problems, such as withdrawal and sadness.

COMMENT

The authors point out that other studies of maltreated children have found an increase in externalizing problems, such as aggression and other disruptive behaviours. They explain that less than 20 per cent of all the children in the study were physically abused, and aggressive behaviour was related to physical abuse but not to neglect.

This study demonstrates the serious damage children suffer when they are neglected and physically abused. Many of these negative effects can affect a child's development and increase their chances of developing psychiatric disorders, such as conduct and depressive disorders. These disorders, in turn, have serious consequences for the child and for society.

SOURCE

Fantuzzo, J.W., Weiss, A.D., Atkins, M., Meyers, R. & Noone, M. (1998). A contextually relevant assessment of the impact of child maltreatment on the social competencies of low-income urban children. *Journal of the American Academy of Child and Adolescent Psychiatry, 37*, 1201–1208.

Child Abuse and Neglect and the Outcomes

Factors in child abuse and neglect

- Four factors combine and interact in child maltreatment (abuse and neglect) and its effects on children's adjustment and psychopathology:
  - individual parents
  - family functioning
  - neighbourhood and social network
  - cultural norms.

- Related factors in child abuse and neglect include stress, unemployment, low socio-economic status, maternal depression, negative life experiences and low marital support. Perhaps the strongest link associated with child maltreatment is poverty:
  - Children in families with incomes under $15,000 were 22 times more likely to experience abuse than those with incomes above $30,000.
  - The most severe cases of maltreatment are linked with the highest levels of poverty.

Individual parents

- Often, parents who maltreat their children are socially isolated from sources of support, have social skill deficits and tend to make hostile attributions (they assume that ambiguous behaviour in others is hostile).

- They often have less information about age-appropriate behaviours, resulting in false expectations and increased frustration.

- They may perceive child-rearing as more difficult and less enjoyable, and report higher associated levels of anger, unhappiness and rigidity than non-maltreating parents.

- Children in single-parent homes are at a 77 per cent greater risk of physical abuse and an 87 per cent greater chance of sexual abuse.

- Single mothers who felt inadequate tended to have negative perceptions of their children.

- Maternal depression is strongly linked to psychiatric disorders in children.

Family functioning

- Research in family functioning has shown that three factors—cohesion, expressiveness and conflict—are related to later child outcomes in abusive families.

- Low cohesion, less parent-child involvement and poor parental supervision of children are linked with conduct disorders, depression and substance use.

- The quality of the parents' relationship affects the child's conduct problems and antisocial behaviour.

- Marital conflict predicts greater adjustment problems in children than does global marital distress (the everyday difficulties common to most marriges).

Outcomes of child abuse and neglect

- Maltreated children are at risk of developing physical and mental health problems and difficulties in acquiring knowledge. Multiple stressors increase the risk: a single stressor led to a one per cent increase, two stressors were linked with a five per cent increase, and four or more stressors led to a 21 per cent increase in subsequent problems.

- Child maltreatment can harm the child's social competence, self-esteem, autonomy, emotional adjustment, school performance and IQ.

- Physically abused children tend to develop insecure attachments as a result of poor, inconsistent care, rejection and harsh interactions. These children respond with more aggression, use less control on their emotions and have depression, delayed social awareness (not aware of the effects of their actions on others) and interpersonal difficulties.

- Sexually abused children may exhibit anxiety, depression, suicidal ideation, sleep complaints, self-destructive behaviour, antisocial behaviour and school problems. Obviously, physical problems can also result from physical and sexual abuse.

- The effects of abuse vary related to the frequency, duration and intensity of the abuse as well as the child's innate resources and environment.

- Chronic adverse conditions and the absence of child supports are associated with problems being passed down from parents to children.

COMMENT

Both the children and the adults who are abusing them should receive treatment once abuse or neglect is identified.

SOURCE

Hecht, D.B. & Hansen, D.J. (2001). The environment of child maltreatment: Contextual factors and the development of psychopathology. *Aggression and Violent Behavior, 6(5)*, 433–457.

Bullying and Its Consequences

Bullying is a form of abuse: it is unprovoked, intentional and its aim is to cause pain and distress to another child. It can be verbal, physical or both. The purpose of this study was to assess bullying and psychological disturbances in 5,813 elementary-school-aged children. Questionnaires were given to parents, teachers and children regarding the children's involvement in bullying (as bullies, bully-victims and victims).

RESULTS

- 8.1 per cent of all children were bullies: 13.3 per cent of boys and 2.8 per cent of girls.

- 7.6 per cent of children were both bullies and victims of bullying: 12.7 per cent of boys and 2.4 per cent of girls.

- 11.3 per cent of children were victims of bullying: 12.8 per cent of boys and 9.7 per cent of girls.

- Children who were involved in bullying were found to have psychological disturbances.

- Surprisingly, the study found bullies and victims to be equally affected by psychological problems.

- Children who were both bullies and victims had the most serious psychological problems. These children showed aggressive behaviour and other externalizing behaviours, including hyperactivity.

- Victims had internalizing problems, such as anxiety and depression.

- It is also possible that depression makes children more prone to be victims of bullying. Studies have shown that victims have low self-esteem, poor problem-solving skills, are immature for their age and are lonely.

- Absenteeism from school may be related to bullying.

COMMENT

The findings in this study are supported by other studies on the subject. The facts that both bullies and victims have psychological disturbances and that very few children involved in bullying are referred for help warrants the concern of parents and teachers.

SOURCE

Kumpulainen, K., Räsänen, E., Irmeli, H., Fredrik, A., Kresanov, K., Linna, S., Moilanen, I., Piha, J., Puura, K. & Tamminen, T. (1998). Bullying and psychiatric symptoms among elementary school-age children. *Child Abuse and Neglect*, 22, 705–717.

Child Neglect, Temperament and Family Context

Studies have indicated that, in areas of social, emotional and academic functioning, children who are neglected do as poorly as children who are abused. Neglect is commonly classified as physical or emotional, or both. Physical neglect is defined as not meeting the child's need for food, clothing, shelter and safety. Emotional neglect is defined as a lack of emotional warmth and responsiveness towards the child.

This study examined the relationship between physical and emotional neglect, temperament and family context. The study included 120 women of low income (77 per cent of these women were receiving Aid to Families with Dependant Children) who had young children averaging about 18 months old.

RESULTS

- Mothers who perceived their children as having an easier temperament had more positive interactions with their children.

- Mothers who were living in more supportive family environments perceived their children more positively.

- Child neglect was less likely if the mother was involved in a positive family situation, which was found to influence her perception of her child's temperament as being relatively easy.

- The child's temperament and family context were not significantly related to physical neglect.

COMMENT

Clinicians should pay attention to how parents describe their child's behaviour (even though it may not be consistent with the reports of teachers or other observers) as this description may provide insight into parenting behaviour. Mothers who experience chronic stress associated with poverty may be unable to separate their child's problem behaviours from their own stress. Studies have shown that focusing only on the child's behaviour is not the best strategy, as parents need and appreciate the attention to their own problems as well.

SOURCE

Harrington, D., Black, M.M., Starr, R.H. & Dubowitz, H. (1998). Child neglect: Relation to child temperament and family context. *American Journal of Orthopsychiatry, 68,* 108–116.

Causes and Contributing Factors

Physical Punishment: What Makes It More or Less Harmful?

Evidence suggests that harsh physical discipline during preschool years increases the chances of the child developing assaultive behaviour in the adolescent years. This study, however, suggests that the relationship between physical punishment and aggression is not that simple. Many factors may increase or decrease physical punishment's harmful effects on behaviour.

RESULTS

Child-parent relationship

- If the parent-child relationship is distant, and the child perceives the parent giving the punishment as uncaring, the effects of the punishment will be severe.

- On the other hand, if the child and parent have a good relationship and the child perceives the parent as loving and caring, the effect of physical punishment may be negligible.

Cultural context

- Studies indicate cultural differences in perceptions of the appropriateness of physical punishment. One study showed that African-American women viewed physical punishment and reasoning as equally appropriate and non-abusive strategies. In contrast, European-American women thought physical punishment was indicative of less positive (defined as concern for the child) and more abusive parenting.

- The authors suggest that, while such results should be interpreted with caution, parental discipline behaviour may be best understood within cultural contexts rather than by relying solely on comparisons between groups.

Gender of parent and child

- There is some evidence that the adverse effects of physical punishment are magnified if the child and the parent are of the same gender (e.g., the father punishing the son). If the child and parent are of different genders, the effects are not as severe.

- This may occur because the child sees a parent of the same gender as more of a role model.

COMMENT

Physical punishment as a method of disciplining children remains common in North America. One survey found that 79 per cent to 97 per cent of three-year-olds are physically punished in any given year and 11 per cent of children experience severe violence that amounts to physical abuse. There is consensus in the literature that physical punishment that meets the definition of physical abuse is always harmful. Even mild, occasional physical punishment carries certain risks. With knowledge of these facts, every effort should be made to convince parents not to use physical punishment, that alternative ways of disciplining children are more effective and carry little risk.

SOURCE

Deater-Deckard, K., Dodge, K.A., Bates, J.E. & Pettit, G.S. (1997). Externalizing behavior problems and discipline revisited: Nonlinear effects and variation by culture, context, and gender. *Psychological Inquiry, 8(3)*, 161–175.

Physical Punishment—When Is It Harmful?

Many studies show that physical punishment of children is harmful and fosters antisocial and aggressive behaviour. This study attempted to overcome some of the methodological difficulties of past research by:

- using a proportional measure of corporal punishment (looking at differences in the results of moderate physical punishment and severe physical punishment)

- taking into account earlier behaviour problems and other dimensions of parenting.

In addition, most of the previous studies have been based on Anglo-American families living in the United States. The authors view this as a major limitation, because the effects of corporal punishment may differ by culture.

This study looked at a sample of Iowa families who used physical punishment moderately and Taiwanese families who used physical punishment severely and frequently.

RESULTS

- There was no evidence of a relationship between physical punishment and behaviour problems in the children of the Iowa families.

- In the Taiwanese families, there was a relationship between physical punishment and behaviour problems, but only when children did not receive any warmth and control from either parent.

COMMENT

The authors note that, while many American families sometimes use corporal punishment to discipline their children, the current evidence does not warrant a view of these parents as misguided or ineffective.

The authors conclude that physical punishment leads to antisocial behaviour only when it is severe or administered in the absence of parental warmth and involvement.

The conclusions that can be drawn are that physical punishment is always harmful when:

- it is severe and is abusive

- it is administered by non-caring, uninvolved parents.

The question is, why should physical punishment be used at all? It is a risky procedure and can be harmful under certain conditions, particularly when it is used out of anger and annoyance. In these cases, the parent is indirectly relaying the message that it is acceptable to hit people in anger. Other consequences—such as time out, loss of privileges, or rewards for good and acceptable behaviour—can improve behaviour when used consistently and do not carry the associated risks that physical punishment does.

SOURCE

Simons, R.L., Wu, C., Lin, K., Gordon, L. & Conger, R.D. (2000). A cross-cultural examination of the link between corporal punishment and adolescent antisocial behavior. *Criminology, 38*, 47–79.

Maltreatment and Abusive Relationships

This study looked at how maltreatment of children before age 12 may affect adolescent peer and dating relationships. Maltreatment in this study was determined through self-reports. The youth reported on experiences of physical or sexual abuse or witnessing violence between their parents. Out of 369 Grade 9 and 10 students, 36 per cent were classified as maltreated and 64 per cent as non-maltreated. There was little difference in percentages of males and females within the two groups.

RESULTS

Results revealed that both males and females who had experienced maltreatment:

- scored high on the measurement of interpersonal sensitivity and hostility, indicating personal inadequacy, inferiority and hostility

- had problems with closeness and trust in intimate relationships

- showed more negative physical and verbal behaviours toward dating partners

- reported being coercive and emotionally abusive toward their dating partner, yet, interestingly, also complained of receiving similar behaviour from their dating partner.

SOURCE

Wolfe, D., Wekerle, C., Reitzel-Jaffe, D. & Lefebvre, L. (1998). Factors associated with abusive relationships among maltreated and non-maltreated youth. *Development and Psychopathology, 10*, 61–85.

Physical and Sexual Abuse and Gang Involvement

Past studies show that childhood maltreatment, including physical and sexual abuse, is linked with antisocial behaviour, eating disorders, teenage pregnancy, substance use and suicide. However, it is not clear whether childhood maltreatment is linked with gang involvement.

This study of 2,468 students, in grades 6 through 12, was designed to determine if maltreatment increases the chances of youth involvement in gangs. The study was conducted using a self-report questionnaire. The students were assured of anonymity. Most students were "white"; Hispanic youth formed the next-largest group.

RESULTS

- 14.5 per cent reported they had been physically abused to the point of injury.

- 8 per cent reported they had been sexually abused. Girls were eight times more likely to have experienced sexual abuse than boys.

- Youth from single-parent families were twice as likely to be physically and sexually abused than youth from two-parent families.

- Black youth and youth of American Indian or Hispanic descent were more likely to be abused than white youth and those of Asian descent.

- 37 per cent of the youth who were physically abused engaged in gang fighting, compared with 20 per cent among those who were not physically abused. Figures for sexual abuse were 32 per cent compared to 21 per cent among the same groups.

- Youth who were abused both physically and sexually were four times more likely to join gangs than those who were not.

- Youth who were abused repeatedly were only slightly more likely to join gangs than those who were abused occasionally. Thus, it is more important to prevent abuse from occurring at all than to intervene after it has occurred.

COMMENT

To explain the link between maltreatment and gang involvement, the authors suggest that young people who are physically abused seek out groups that use similar methods of resolving disputes.

This study indicates that youth from single-parent homes and those from "non-white" families (e.g., American Indian, Hispanic and Black) were more likely to be physically and sexually abused. It has to be remembered that these groups are more likely to belong to lower income groups, and poverty is associated with both physical and mental problems in families.

SOURCE

Thompson, K.M. & Braaten-Antrim, R. (1998). Youth maltreatment and gang involvement. *Journal of Interpersonal Violence, 13*, 328–345.

Prevention

Unskilled Disciplining of Children and Abuse

This study illustrates that parents who are unskilled in disciplining their children can create an environment in the home where child abuse, neglectful supervision and sibling conflict occurs.

RESULTS

- Child maltreatment was a significant predictor of antisocial behaviour, accidents, injuries and illness, arrests for violent crime and physical aggression to partners.

- Neglectful supervision was a significant predictor of poor academic performance, antisocial behaviour, association with troubled peers, accidents, injuries and illness.

- Sibling conflict was a significant predictor of antisocial behaviour, substance use and arrests for violent crime.

- The impact of unskilled discipline practices and the consequent abusive home environment can predict a variety of adjustment outcomes as children move into adolescence and early adulthood.

COMMENT

The authors suggest that interventions to improve discipline practices will also reduce abusive and neglectful practices in the home environment.

Giving parents courses on sound childrearing practices can help prevent the development of many disorders in children—disorders that result from unskilled discipline and abuse and have serious consequences in adolescence and adulthood.

SOURCE

Bank, L. & Burraston, B. (2001). Abusive home environments as predictors of poor adjustment during adolescence and early adulthood. *Journal of Community Psychology, 29(3)*, 195–217.

Preventing Child Abuse and Neglect

This article outlines two basic approaches to preventing child abuse and neglect. Both approaches include services to families who are at high risk, such as low-income families, and households with young mothers or unwanted pregnancy.

The approaches to preventing maltreatment involve programs that:

* support parents and families with services such as quality childcare, parenting programs, decent housing, mental health services for parents and children

* involve home visiting by nurses, professionals or trained volunteers— evidence indicates that home visiting can prevent childhood injuries and reduce abuse and neglect.

To be effective, these programs must begin early, happen often and extend over the first few years of a child's life.

SOURCE

Leventhal, J. (1997). The prevention of child abuse and neglect: Pipe dreams or possibilities? *Clinical Child Psychology and Psychiatry, 2*, 489–500.

Treatment

Treatment for the Long-Term Effects of Child Abuse

This was a review of studies published on the long-term consequences of child abuse (including physical abuse, sexual abuse and neglect).

RESULTS

- Abused children are at risk of long-term psychological problems related to the abuse itself, not only as a consequence of associated background factors (e.g., punitive parenting styles, social disadvantage, physical unattractiveness).

- The type of abuse experienced is somewhat related to the type of psychological outcome. For example, victims of sexual abuse often feel stigma and blame.

- Physical abuse is just as traumatic as sexual abuse in the long-term.

- Most of the adverse psychological problems can also arise in the absence of abuse (i.e., aggression and depression). There are few signs specific only to abuse.

- An important feature affecting both short- and long-term outcomes is adequate resolution of child protection issues and the prevention of further abuse.

- No matter how effective specific psychological treatments are, broad service measures, such as good housing, adequate financial support and affordable, quality daycare, can help parents better care for their children, which may in turn help to prevent abuse and maltreatment.

- In general, psychological treatments are about as effective for children as they are for adults.

- There are few well-conducted and adequately controlled studies of the effectiveness of treatment for children who have been abused.

- Some areas have been studied extensively (e.g., group therapy for sexually abused children). From these studies, it appears that treatment for children who have been abused is as effective as for children whose problems arise from other causes.

- Training can change parenting.

- A substantial number (a minority) of abused children do not show symptoms related to their abuse.

- Planning services for the long-term effects of abuse must account for the needs of survivors of abuse in adulthood, when disclosure may occur for the first time.

COMMENT

The authors suggest that physical abuse is just as traumatic as sexual abuse in the long-term; however, it is hard to quantitatively measure how traumatic abuse is in the long-term.

It is important to consider specific concerns relevant to different types of abuse. For example, one study found that sexual abuse carried the greatest risk of attempted suicide. In addition, sexual abuse carries with it feelings of stigma and blame that are both internalized (e.g., through depression and feelings of worthlessness) and externalized (e.g., acting out, attempting suicide).

SOURCE

Stevenson, J. (1999). The treatment of the long-term sequelae of child abuse. *Journal of Child Psychology and Psychiatry, 40,* 89–111.

Chapter 7
Substance
Related Disorders

Substance Related Disorders

A cluster of cognitive, behavioural and
physiological symptoms indicating
that the individual continues to use
the substance despite significant
substance-related problems.

Characteristics and Related Issues

Substance Use Problems in Adolescents Receiving Care

A recent community sample estimated 6.2 per cent of the young people had substance use disorder (SUD). This study examined the prevalence of substance use disorder in youth receiving public services in the following five sectors of care: alcohol and drug treatment, juvenile justice system, mental health care, school-based services for youths with serious emotional disturbance and child welfare services.

RESULTS

* Youth with SUD were identified in all five sectors. However, the rates of SUD differed markedly between sectors:
  - alcohol and drug treatment, 82.6 per cent
  - juvenile justice system, 62.1 per cent
  - mental health care, 40.8 per cent
  - school-based services, 23.6 per cent
  - child welfare services, 19.2 per cent.

COMMENT

The authors suggest that professionals should be sensitive to the likelihood of substance use disorder not only in settings providing substance use treatment but also in all settings providing care for young people.

SOURCE

Aarons, G.A., Brown, S.A., Hough, R.L., Garland, A.F. & Wood, P.A. (2001). Prevalence of adolescent substance use disorders across five sectors of care. *Journal of the American Academy of Child and Adolescent Psychiatry, 40(4),* 419–426.

Behaviour Problems and Marijuana Use

RESULTS

* Young people who have conduct problems in their early teens are at high risk of using marijuana in adolescence.

- Although conduct problems are less common among girls, girls with conduct problems have a greater risk of using marijuana than boys with conduct disorders.

- Cigarette smoking appears to be an important precursor to marijuana use.

COMMENT

This study was done in Norway during the early 1990s, but the association between substance use and behaviour problems was also true in North America. However, the authors question whether the results are still valid in today's society, when the use of marijuana is becoming more the norm in youth culture.

SOURCE

Pederson, W., Mastekaasa, A. & Wichstrom, L. (2001). Conduct problems and early cannabis initiation: A longitudinal study of gender differences. *Addiction, 96(3)*, 415–431.

Drug Use in Girls

Drug use has increased significantly in girls during the past 30 years. Throughout the 1960s, only 5 per cent of girls between ages 10 and 14 used marijuana, compared to 24 per cent in the 1990s. Moreover, there is no longer a difference in frequency of drug use between girls and boys.

This study is based on youth referred to a drug treatment program.

RESULTS

- The girls used drugs as often as the boys.

- The girls engaged in antisocial behaviour as often as the boys.

- The girls had more internalizing symptoms, such as depression and anxiety.

- The girls referred to the drug treatment program came from families that were more dysfunctional than the boys' families.

COMMENT

In treating girls for drug use problems, the authors suggest attention both to treating the internalizing symptoms and to treating the malfunctioning family systems.

SOURCE

Dakof, G.A. (2000). Understanding gender differences in adolescent drug abuse: Issues of comorbidity and family functioning. *Journal of Psychoactive Drugs, 32,* 25–32.

Chapter 8
Suicide

Suicide

The act or incidence of taking one's own
life voluntarily and intentionally. Suicidal
behaviour includes suicidal ideation
(thinking about, or planning, suicide)
and suicide attempt.

Characteristics and Related Issues

Suicide in Young Adolescents

Suicide is less common in younger adolescents than in older adolescents. There are also fewer warning signs and precipitating events for suicide among younger adolescents than for older adolescents.

The purpose of this study was to examine the characteristics and risk factors that contribute to the greater incidence of suicide in older adolescents compared to younger adolescents. The study compared two groups of children who had committed suicide: 14 children under the age of 15 and 115 adolescents between the ages of 15 and 19.

RESULTS

- Among precipitating events, younger children often had conflicts with parents, whereas older adolescents more often had conflicts with peers (e.g., romantic disappointment).

- Among psychiatric disorders, affective disorders (e.g., depression) were more common in older adolescents than younger adolescents.

- Both groups had similar levels of disruptive disorders: older adolescents at 14 per cent versus younger adolescents at 10 percent.

COMMENT

The authors conclude that when depression and other risk factors are detected, younger adolescents may be as likely as older adolescents to commit suicide. However, suicide in younger adolescents remains less frequent and less predictable. Therefore, developing prevention programs for younger adolescents presents a great challenge.

SOURCE

Groholt, B., Ekeberg, O., Wichstrom, L. & Haldorsen, T. (1998). Suicide among children and younger and older adolescents in Norway: A comparative study. *Journal of the American Academy of Child and Adolescent Psychiatry, 37*, 473–481.

Suicidal Thoughts and Behaviours among Adolescents

The frequency of suicidal attempts increases sharply during the adolescent years. This increase may be due to developmental stresses and physical, psychological and increased social pressures.

RESULTS

- This study showed that at age 16, 14 per cent of girls and 7 per cent of boys reported suicidal thoughts or preoccupations.

- Internalizing problems (depression), externalizing problems (antisocial behaviours) and social incompetence were associated with suicidal features (suicidal thoughts and attempts).

- Almost three times as many adolescents reported suicidal features than their parents had observed, and only 20 per cent of adolescents who reported suicidal features were referred to mental health services.

COMMENT

Emotional and behavioural problems reported by parents and teachers when children were eight years old were associated with suicidal tendencies eight years later. Thus, intervention during early school years may prevent self-destructive behaviour in adolescence.

SOURCE

Sourander, A., Helstela, L., Haavisto, A. & Bergroth, L. (2001). Suicidal thoughts and attempts among adolescents: A longitudinal 8-year follow-up study. *Journal of Affective Disorders, 63(1–3)*, 59–66.

Suicide in Adolescents with Disruptive Disorders

Past studies have associated conduct disorder with suicide, especially for people who also have mood disorder and substance use problems. The objective of this study was to determine which factors distinguish youth with disruptive behaviour disorders (i.e., conduct disorder, oppositional defiant disorder and attention-deficit hyperactivity disorder) who commit suicide from those who do not.

RESULTS

Youth with conduct disorder who committed suicide differed from youth with conduct disorder who did not commit suicide in the following areas (the numbers are presented respectively):

- current substance abuse (45.6 per cent versus 5.6 per cent)
- lifetime physical abuse (55.2 per cent versus 0 per cent)
- past suicide attempts (52.7 per cent versus 5.6 per cent)
- suicidal ideation (52.5 per cent versus 16.7 per cent)
- family history of substance abuse (23.9 per cent versus 4.1 per cent)
- family history of affective disorder (27.6 per cent versus 14 per cent).

COMMENT

Unlike other studies, the results of this study did not show that the presence of a major affective disorder with a disruptive disorder increased the risk of suicide. The study did indicate, however, that youth with conduct disorder were more likely to commit suicide than youth with ADHD.

It should be noted that one of the strongest factors that differentiated youth who committed suicide from those who did not was a history of lifetime physical abuse. This is important, as many parents continue to use physical punishment and believe it is harmless.

SOURCE

Renaud, J., Brent, D.A. & Birmaher, B. (1999). Suicide in adolescents with disruptive disorders. *Journal of the American Academy of Child and Adolescent Psychiatry, 38,* 846–851.

Homicide-Suicide and Other Forms of Aggression

Of all psychiatric emergency service visits, about 20 per cent are related to suicidal risk and 10 to 17 per cent are related to homicidal risk. Assessing the risk of harm to self (suicide) and the risk of harm to others (homicide) are distinct clinical processes. However, these forms of aggression often coexist (e.g., homicide-suicide, where one or more homicides is followed by the perpetrator's suicide). Studies show a strong link between these two forms of aggression, suggesting that risk assessment should include the risk for both conditions of suicide and homicide. Several models explain the interaction:

Countervailing factors

- Losses, threats, challenges and status changes increase aggressive impulses, while criticism or rejection activates them.

- Distrust, access to weapons and a tolerant attitude toward aggression increase the likelihood of activating aggressive impulses.

- Timidity, close family ties and appeasement from others decrease aggressive impulses.

- Hopelessness and depression increase the probability of self-harm.

- Impulsivity, conduct disorder and mental illness increase the likelihood of aggression against others.

- A person who has both hopelessness and impulsivity would be at an increased risk of co-occurring aggression against self and others.

Biopsychosocial factors

- Serotonin is a chemical in the body that is known to be involved in behavioural inhibition. Dysfunction in the serotonin system is suspected to be involved in aggression against self and others. A person with dysfunction in the serotonin system will be more sensitive to stimuli that elicit aggression and less sensitive to cues that signal punishment.

- Psychological factors include modelling (observing suicidal behaviour in family members or friends), negative emotions, depression, hopelessness and despair, negative or positive reinforcement, command hallucinations (hallucinations that suggest suicidal behaviour), impulsivity, problem substance use and anger.

- Social factors include exposure to media reports of violence or suicide, access to firearms, poor social supports, unemployment and cultural factors.

Cognitive perspective

- The same cognitive distortions play a large role in causing violence against self (suicide) and violence against others: automatic thoughts, catastrophizing, black-and-white thinking and taking all events personally. The sequence is as follows: loss and fear, distress, focus on the offender, feelings of anger, mobilization for attack.

- Externally directed aggression involves a focus on the person perceived to be causing the distress whereas self-directed aggression does not.

IMPLICATIONS

Risk for threat of suicide or homicide should be assessed at the same time, using current guidelines for both.

Evaluations should explore the current crisis, assess for mental illness and substance use, record detailed history of any past acts of harm against self or others (ideally independently corroborated) and current stressors (interpersonal, occupational, financial, medical, legal, social, existential, spiritual).

Support systems, deterrents to aggression, availability of weapons or lethal martial arts techniques, and past response and adherence to treatment are also assessed.

Protective factors to review include intelligence, spiritual beliefs, reasons for living, positive social orientation, resilient temperament, healthy beliefs about achievement and supportive relationships.

It is important to determine if there was a history of disruptive behaviour in childhood and adolescence and if depression coexisted with violent behaviour and a lifelong pattern of quick temper, impulsivity, problem substance use and interpersonal difficulties. To date, this is the only developmental pathway that has been associated with co-occurring aggression against others and against self (homicide-suicide).

TREATMENT

Treatments for threat of suicide or violence share an overall strategy:

- Reduce risk factors.
- Increase barriers to aggression.
- Treat associated disorders.

Treatment for risk of harm to self includes:

- medications
- environmental manipulations
- social and family supports
- altering negative thinking patterns

- substance abuse management
- limiting access to lethal means
- hospitalization for psychiatric treatment.

Treatment for risk of violence to others includes:

- anger and stress management
- anticonvulsant medication
- substance abuse management
- criminal justice intervention (restraining orders, probation, limiting access to weapons, and monitoring).

COMMENT

Depression is the leading risk factor for threat of both suicide and homicide-suicide. Depression is common among people who are violent but is not often mentioned as a treatment target in this population. Similarly, problems managing anger are common among people who are suicidal.

As the serotonergic system is implicated in the causes of depression and aggression, antidepressants (SSRIs) may be indicated in co-occurring aggression against self and against others.

SOURCE

Hillbrand, M. (2001). Homicide-suicide and other forms of co-occurring aggression against self and against others. *Professional Psychology—Research and Practice, 32(6)*, 626–635.

Causes and Contributing Factors

Suicide of Children and Divorce

This study compared the family backgrounds of 120 youth who committed suicide, with a control group of 147 youth, matched in age, gender and ethnicity.

RESULTS

- There was no difference in family structure between the two groups.

- Suicide victims were less likely to be living with their parent(s) at the time of their death. Most of them were living with another relative.

- Suicide victims were more likely to have poor relationships with their fathers, regardless of whether the parents were separated or divorced or not.

- Separation and divorce increased the risk of suicide only when communication was poor with the parents.

COMMENT

The authors conclude that the increase in adolescent suicide cannot be attributed to the increase in the rate of divorce over the last few decades. Instead, some important factors that contribute to suicide among youth are parental mental health and the quality of the father-child relationship.

SOURCE

Gould, M.S., Shaffer, D., Fisher, P. & Garfinkel, R. (1998). Separation/divorce and child and adolescent completed suicide. *Journal of the American Academy of Child and Adolescent Psychiatry, 37,* 155–162.

Psychiatric Contacts and Suicide Attempts

Two models have generally been used to explain the occurrence of suicidal behaviour.

- One model implies that suicide attempts may occur in any person who faces seemingly insurmountable life stresses and sees suicide as the only solution.

- The other model is the mental illness model, which argues that those most at risk for suicidal behaviour are young people with recognizable mental disorders.

The psychiatric histories of 129 young people who made serious suicide attempts were compared to a group of 153 people in community controls to determine which model was more accurate.

RESULTS

- Results indicated that, of those who made suicide attempts, 89 per cent met criteria for a psychiatric disorder, and 80 per cent had previous contact with psychiatric services.

- In comparison with the control group, those making serious suicide attempts had higher rates of:
  - psychiatric hospital admission
  - outpatient psychiatric consultation
  - attendance at support groups for those with mental health problems
  - telephone calls to counselling or crisis helplines.

COMMENT

These findings are consistent with previous studies, which have generally found that between one-third and three-quarters of young people with suicidal behaviour have histories of prior contact with psychiatric services. This indicates that those most at risk for suicidal behaviour are young people with recognizable mental disorders.

IMPLICATIONS

The findings from this study suggest that suicide prevention strategies should clearly identify treatment and management strategies for young people with psychiatric disorders.

SOURCE

Beautrais, A.L., Joyce, P.R. & Mulder, R.T. (1998). Psychiatric contacts among youths aged 13 through 24 years who have made serious suicide attempts. *Journal of the American Academy of Child and Adolescent Psychiatry*, *37*, 504–511.

Youth Victimization, Suicide and Violence

Research indicates that the greatest threat to adolescents' health is their own behaviour. Interpersonal violence has increased by 27 per cent among youths aged 16 to 19 and is responsible for many fatal and non-fatal injuries among adolescents. Suicide is the third leading cause of death among adolescents and young adults, and has increased by 35 per cent among those aged 15 to 19.

The objective of this study was to investigate the associations between peer victimization and the risk of suicidal and violence-related behaviours among 1,569 public high-school students in New York State. The students had previously participated in a youth risk behaviour survey in 1997 and were divided into four groups based on their responses:

- no suicide or violent behaviour
- suicidal behaviour only
- violent behaviour only
- both suicidal and violent behaviour.

Two hypotheses were tested in this study:

- Victimized students would report more suicidal and/or violent behaviour compared with non-victimized students.
- Relationships would vary by gender for victimized students. Specifically, victimized females were expected to report more suicidal behaviours and victimized males were expected to report more violent behaviours.

RESULTS

- 35 per cent of students reported being victimized.
- 49 per cent reported no suicidal or violent behaviour.
- 12 per cent reported suicidal behaviour only.
- 28 per cent reported violent behaviour only.
- 11 per cent reported both suicidal and violent behaviours.
- The risk of violent or suicidal behaviours was 1.4 to 2.6 times greater among victimized students compared with non-victimized students.
- Males reported significantly more victimization, less suicidal behaviour and more violent behaviour than females.
- Females were more likely to report more suicidal behaviour only, whereas males were more likely to report violent behaviour only.

COMMENTS

These findings support both the first hypothesis, which suggested that victimized students would be at greater risk for suicidal and/or violent behaviour, and the second hypothesis, which suggested that behavioural patterns would vary by gender. The study concluded that to reduce inter-personal violence in high schools, components of violence prevention programs should aim to be gender specific. It also concluded that an integral part of comprehensive intervention programs should be to identify and treat victims of violence.

Source

Cleary, S.D. (2000). Adolescent victimization and associated suicidal and violent behaviors. *Adolescence, 35(140)*, 671–682.

Youth Suicidal Ideation, Attempts and Risk Factors

This study examined the relationship between suicidal ideation or attempts with family environment, youth characteristics and various risk behaviours among 1,285 children and adolescents between the ages of nine and 17.

Results

Familial factors significantly associated with suicidal ideation and behaviour include:

- difficult family circumstances
- low satisfaction with the family environment
- low parental monitoring
- parental history of psychiatric disorder.

Factors associated with likelihood of suicidal ideation or behaviour include:

- youth characteristics such as low social and instrumental competence (ability to follow directions, figure out answers in school).

Risk factors that significantly increased the risk for suicidal ideation or attempts include:

- smoking
- physical fighting
- alcohol intoxication
- marijuana
- sexual activity.

SOURCE

King, R.A., Schwab-Stone, M., Flisher, A.J., Greenwald, S., Kramer, R.A., Goodman, S.H., Lahey, B.B., Shaffer, D. & Gould, M.S. (2001). Psychosocial and risk behavior correlates of youth suicide attempts and suicidal ideation. *Journal of the American Academy of Child and Adolescent Psychiatry, 40(7),* 837–846.

Indexes

Author Index

Dowdney, L., 26
Doyle, A., 133
Drinkwater, M., 160
Dubowitz, H., 177
Duncan, S.C., 34
Duncan, T.E., 34
DuPaul, G.J., 129, 141
Duxbury, E., 152

Eckenrode, J., 109
Eckenrode, J.J., 43
Eckert, T.L., 129
Eddy, J.M., 29
Edwards, J., 55
Egeland, B., 22
Ekeberg, O., 195
Espelage, D.L., 20
Eyberg, S.M., 119

Fagot, B.I., 35
Fantuzzo, J.W., 172
Faraone, S.V., 133
Farrell, A.D., 9
Farrington, D.P., v, 16, 157, 161
Feil, E.G., 46
Feldman, S.S., 149
Fergusson, D.M., 15, 31, 32
Finkelhor, D., 11
Fisher, P., 201
Fitzpatrick, K.M., 68
Fitzpatrick, T.M., 54
Flannery, D.J., 4
Fleck, S., 77
Flisher, A.J., 205
Frazier, E., 133
Fredrik, A., 176
Freudenberg, N., 7
Frick, P., 129
Frick, P.J., 90, 99, 98
Frierson, T., 19

Garfinkel, R., 201
Garland, A.F., 189
Gaub, M., 124

Ge, X.J., 71
Gendreau, P.L., 72
Gibbons, R.D., 86
Gillberg, C., 127
Gjone, H., 13
Golly, A., 46
Goodman, S.H., 205
Gordon, L., 180
Gordon, R.A., 157
Gottfredson, D.C., 48
Gould, M.S., 205
Greenberg, M.T., 26
Greene, M.B., 7
Green, S., 129
Green, S.M., 90, 92
Greenwald, S., 205
Groholt, B., 195
Gruber, R., 130
Gullion, M.E., 101

Haapasalo, J., 18
Haavisto, A., 196
Haldorsen, T., 195
Hamburger, S.D., 131
Hammond, M., 92, 114
Hamre, B.K., 59
Hand, L.D., 55
Hansen, D.J., 174
Hanson, R.F., 41
Harrington, D., 177
Harrison, R.J., 69
Hecht, D.B., 174
Helstela, L., 196
Henderson, C.R, 109
Henderson, Jr., C.R., 43
Henggeler, S.W., 44, 55, 78
Heptinstall, E., 97
Hillbrand, M., 200
Hoffman, J.B., 141
Hopkins, J., 16
Hops, H., 34
Horwood, J.L., 15
Horwood, L.J., 31
Hough, R.L., 189

Subject Index

substance use and, 189
treatment, 47, 48, 135, 179
binge drinking, 6
bipolar disorder. *See also* mania;
    mood disorders
    ADHD and, 125–126
    impulsivity and, 23
Black. *See* African-American
boot camps, 76, 164
borderline personality disorder, 23
boys
    ADHD and, 89, 127, 130, 132.
        See also ADHD
    aggression and, 74. *See also*
        aggression
    anger and, 105. *See also* anger
    anxiety and, 88. *See also* mental
        health problems
    bullying and, 4, 175. *See also*
        bullying
    conduct disorders and, 156.
        See also conduct disorder
    crime victimization and, 10
    criminality and, 149
    development of antisocial
        behaviour in, 150, 155
    deviant peers, role of and, 72
    disruptive behaviour and, 31, 85,
        86, 132
    exposure to violence and, 6
    family influence on, 72, 127–128,
        154,
    gangs and, 154, 155–157
    hyperactivity and, 149, 150
    marijuana use by, 189. *See also*
        substance use
    physical assaults and, 68
    physical punishment and, 158
    programs for, 53, 79, 105
    reading disability in, 24, 96
    sleep patterns of, 129–130
    suicide and, 196
    temperament in, 13
Brain Power program, 106

Bry's behaviourally-based
    prevention program, 48
bullying
    access to guns and, 20
    by boys, 4
    bully/victims, 4, 19, 175
    by girls, 4
    contributing social factors, 20
    defined, 20
    direct, 18–19
    effect on children's behaviour, 18,
        34
    effect of parents on, 20
    exposure to violence and, 20
    factors contributing to, 20–21, 175
    frequency of, 20
    illegal activities and, 20
    peer relationships and, 20
    prevention programs for, 77
    primary school children and,
        18–19
    as proactive aggression, 72
    relational, 18–19
    victims of, 4, 19, 34, 175
buspirone, for ADHD, 142

Cambridge-Somerville youth study,
    49
Carey Infant Temperament
    Questionnaire, 38
Caucasian youth, 41, 95
Child Behaviour Checklist, 8, 12, 38,
    39, 52
child abuse. *See also* abuse; bullying;
    neglect; sexual abuse
    consequences of, 108, 170, 174,
        180, 183
    four main factors in, 172
    nurse visitation programs and,
        108
    preventing, 182–183
    related factors in, 173
    sexual, 170, 175
    violence and, 41, 64

restraint and criminal behaviour, 151
rewards, 114
Ritalin. *See* methylphenidate
role-playing, 77, 106, 114
rules, 66, 77, 85, 161

safety, feelings of, 5
schizophrenia-spectrum disorder
 and violence, 63
school-based interventions, 47–48
 for ADHD, 138, 140
 Adolescent Transition Program
  (ATP), 57
 cognitive-behavioural, 56
 for conduct disorder, 101
 Peacemakers, 78
schools
 drug prevention programs in, 77
 environment and aggressive
  behaviour, 67
 family resource rooms in, 58
 preventing antisocial behaviour
  in, 45
 rules in, 67
 services for youth, 189
 shootings, 73
 success determinants in, 59
 teaching social skills, 106
 violence prevention programs in,
  77
screening procedures, 46
Seattle Social Development Project,
 100
Second Step program, 104
selective intervention program, 45,
 105
self-control and preventing violence,
 66
self-esteem
 child maltreatment and, 169
 gang entry and, 155
 low, and delinquency, 51
 value of promoting, 55
self-injury, 68. *See also* suicide

self-report measures, 23
serotonin, 198
sexual abuse
 adolescent sex offences and, 162
 behaviour problems and, 31
 dissociative disorders and, 65
 effects of, 162
 family dysfunction and, 171
 feelings of blame and, 183
 gang involvement and, 181
 as predictor for sexual offending,
  52, 162
 single-parent family and, 173, 181
 treatment programs for child
  victims, 169, 174
sexual activity, as risk factor
 for suicide, 204
sexual assault, higher-income
 households, 41
sexual interest, as predictor of sexual
 offences, 51
sexual offences
 predicting, 51
 treatment programs for, 51
sibling conflict, and antisocial
 behaviour, 182
single-parent family
 antisocial behaviour and, 22, 158
 conduct disorder and, 108
 physical abuse, risk of in, 173, 181
 sexual abuse, risk of in, 173, 181
skills, teaching effective, 45
sleep
 ADHD and, 129–130
 exposure to violence and, 9
small-group interventions, for
 aggressive behaviour, 105
smoking
 behaviour problems and, 31
 peer interventions and, 58
 prevention programs for, 47
 suicide and, 204
social competence, 100, 174
social exclusion, 20